Methodology for the Observation of Hidden Behaviours in Addiction

Methodology for the Observation of Hidden Behaviours in Addiction

By

Casimiro Balsa, Cláudia Urbano
and Clara Vital

Translated by Alison Roberts

Cambridge
Scholars
Publishing

Methodology for the Observation of Hidden Behaviours in Addiction

By Casimiro Balsa, Cláudia Urbano and Clara Vital

This book first published 2023

Cambridge Scholars Publishing

Lady Stephenson Library, Newcastle upon Tyne, NE6 2PA, UK

British Library Cataloguing in Publication Data
A catalogue record for this book is available from the British Library

ISBN (10): 1-5275-3192-9
ISBN (13): 978-1-5275-3192-5

TABLE OF CONTENTS

Index of Figures

INDEX OF TABLES

General Introduction

This work is part of a broader project aimed at systematising a great deal of information scattered across a series of technical reports produced over a period of 20 years, as part of Portugal's national survey on drug use among general population (INPG — *Inquérito Nacional ao Consumo de Substâncias Psicoativas na População Geral, Portugal*).

After the publication of our study on alcohol and drug use by the working population (Balsa, Urbano and Vital 2021), it is now time to focus on discussion of the more methodological aspects involved in a study of this nature. In a forthcoming volume, we will systematise alcohol and drug use trends in Portugal over the last 20 years.

We propose to organise this discussion in four parts:

We shall begin by discussing the difficulties presented by a study that, in addition to having behaviour that is hidden as an object of observation, must also deal with the strategies of drug users who have every reason to conceal a censored behaviour from an interviewer who knocks on their door. Control procedures will be discussed that seek to guarantee the validity and reliability of the results obtained.

In the second part, we shall discuss the effect of information collection techniques on the results obtained. Once the option is made to conduct face-to-face interviews—which is difficult as well as expensive—the question is to know how the results would have been different if we had used more affordable techniques, such as a telephone or internet survey.

In the third part, we shall try to better elucidate the question of measuring the use, particularly of alcohol, which is, after all, the primary objective of the bodies promoting the study. Despite the importance of this question, it has not been easy to harmonise the measures between the different sources of information.

Finally, we shall make a technical presentation of the methodology of the national survey on drug use among general population.

A work of this nature necessarily involves the participation of many institutions and people working not only in the field of science but also in the areas of the conception, organisation and intervention relating to the various aspects of the problems associated with consumption, whether in prevention and dissuasion, risk reduction and the minimisation of harms when consumption occurs, or in the treatment of addicts and their reintegration into society.

In the first instance, the national survey on drug use among general population should be set within the framework of the policies promoted by the European Union and managed by the European Monitoring Centre for Drugs and Drug Addiction. But it is above all important to anchor it at national level, as a tool to support decision making, within the scope of Portugal's policy on the decriminalisation of drug use. SICAD — the General Directorate for Intervention on Addictive Behaviours and Dependencies — plays an important role here, as do the bodies that preceded it with a similar function: for example, the Office for Planning and Coordination of the Fight Against Drugs, of which Dr Joaquim Rodrigues was Director General (and a member of the commission that defined the first National Strategy for the Fight Against Drugs, as was Dr João Goulão, currently SICAD's Director General). We would like to thank, in the persons of these two officials—Dr Rodrigues, who entrusted us with the task of carrying out the first INPG, and Dr João Goulão, who has maintained that confidence—all the staff of the institution for all the professional, open and always friendly cooperation we have enjoyed over these years.

On the scientific level, we recall the lessons we learned back in the 1990s within the Pompidou Group; in particular, we remember Richard Hartnoll. Later, we also benefited from the expertise and friendship of François Beck and the support of France's Monitoring Centre for Drugs and Drug Addiction (OFDT). The friendship and expertise of Jacinto Osuna Rodriguez and the sharing of his experience in the design and organisation of samples in Spain's national survey were indispensable. To Luís Fernandes, our esteemed colleague from the The Faculty of Psychology and Educational Sciences of the University of Porto, we also express our thanks for the exchanges in our series of interdisciplinary meetings "Olhares Cruzados sobre as Drogas" and other opportunities for fruitful comparisons.

Along the way in these 20 years, all the researchers and employees of NOVA FCSH who at one time or another worked on the team and contributed to the results that we present here were of equal importance:

Miguel Chaves, João Pedro Nunes, Tiago Farinha, André Francisco and Liliana Pascueiro, as well as Cláudia Urbano, from the beginning, and Clara Vital, since the application of the Survey in 2007, who share the authorship of this work. Thanks also go to Paula Bouça, who acted as secretary to the team for many years and whom we have missed greatly since her well-earned retirement.

We would also like to thank the experts at SICAD for their critical and essential review of the manuscript. If any of their suggestions for development fell short of what was expected, this is due to our own limitations.

Finally, a word of thanks to the data collection company, Intercampus, which has provided us with its valuable and professional help from the beginning, and whose work has served to lend credibility to our results.

PART I

OPACITY OF INFORMATION, DISSIMULATION OF BEHAVIOURS AND RECONFIGURATION OF POPULATION OBSERVED: VALIDITY AND RELIABILITY OF SURVEYS ON DRUG USE IN THE GENERAL POPULATION

Presentation

Framework of information analysed and objectives

In this first part of the study, we propose to discuss some of the issues that arise between the design and application of a questionnaire aimed at amassing knowledge about hidden behaviours that, in this case, manifest themselves around the use of psychoactive substances, especially when we consider that these behaviours are subject to greater censorship by dominant norms. We are not interested, for now, in focusing on the multiple technical difficulties presented in designing a questionnaire that has to take into account profiles of very diverse and socially very dense situations, nor the difficulties posed by the construction of a representative sample at national level, when there are no reliable survey bases, nor even the difficulties of programming and carrying out a face-to-face interview in the field with a sample that has varied between 12,000 and 15,000 individuals[1]. What does interest us is discussing the possibility and the conditions of viability of the field work and the degree of confidence that can be attributed to the information collected, when we aim to study hidden behaviours such as those that characterise, to a greater or lesser extent and depending on the circumstances, the use of psychoactive substances, especially illicit ones[2].

---

[1] These questions will be discussed in Part III.

[2] A conference that we organised in 2005 on hidden behaviours began a train of reflection whose first results were published in 2019 (Balsa 2019).

The question arises here in a totally different way from the one we face when we hope to reduce the opacity with which other research objects present themselves. In fact, most commonly, we can consider that difficulties in observation are to be found more on the side of the researcher and their research instruments, when faced with the distance that always inserts itself between the observable and the observed. This distance, due to the complexity that generally characterises the objects of observation, and contrary to the positivist ideal, is difficult to overcome. In the case of the study of drug use, in addition to this usual opacity, researchers must face the difficulties that arise from the fact that the populations and behaviours observed hide themselves from the observer's gaze.

How, then, can the researcher study these behaviours or populations that are hidden? Moreover, with what legitimacy can he do so, since this places him in a situation that breaks the codes of social relations, as conventionally arranged, because by definition what is hidden is what one does not want to or cannot show. Several questions may be posed here. What, after all, is hidden and to what extent does one want to hide it? Between the fully transparent and the fully hidden, might there not be a more or less wide range of intermediate positions? From whom is it hidden and who can know? In what circumstances can this happen? It sometimes happens that individuals hide their consumption from themselves... so why should they declare it to anyone else? Individuals almost always define the boundaries between those who can and those who cannot know, taking into account the type of normative control or elective affinities that mark the meaning of relationships. In some cases, the circumstances of their consumption mean that they can no longer hide. There are far fewer cases in which consumption is presented explicitly as a way of life.

We may think that, through the different positions that drug users take, the last entities to know are those most easily associated with a censorious, if not punitive, normative framework, including official bodies. Under these circumstances, it is worth asking what the fate will be of a researcher's door-to-door questionnaire to find out whether people "use drugs".

What is hidden is thus a status relative to behaviour, but it targets only those of whom it is considered that they cannot or should not see something. In fact, it is on the basis of this assumption that a space opens up for research to construct its strategies of unveiling. The knowledge obtained through these strategies thus demands the clarification on the one hand of the determinations of the gaze of those who hide (but, after all, how to know who hides and what is hidden?) and, on the other, of the limits of the instruments of observation that aim to unveil them.

Moreover, the knowledge that is strategically constructed in this way will enter into competition with other knowledge, supported by the most diverse points of view, that reduces the "realities" about consumption, increasing its opacity. In this way, for example, a municipal official may think that the prevalence rates of consumption that we calculate understate reality, because he is thinking of that neighbourhood "full of drug addicts" that he knows. Similarly, another will tell us that the results are inflated in relation to what he "sees". This construction of "reality", which allows multiple representations about the extent of drug use, can even be observed in professional circles: before our first estimate of the prevalence of illicit substance use in Portugal was known, the expectations of those working in the field with whom we discussed it were divided as to whether it would be below, at the level of, or above the European average...

Our challenges therefore present themselves between opacity and dissimulation. On the one hand, it is a question of acknowledging and making explicit the limits of the capacity to see inherent in the observation functions that the researcher constructs. Yes, that he "constructs", because rather than simply "using" instruments or following such and such a procedure, the researcher is ultimately always the producer and the only one responsible for the research functions to which he may resort, even the most canonical ones, because he will always have to adapt them to "his hand" (much more than to his "measure"). On the other hand, neither the decision to dissimulate nor the dissimulation strategies that constitute obstacles to the researcher's capacity to see can be ignored. It is probable that this confrontation between, on the one hand, opacity and dissimulation and, on the other, the strategies of unveiling that aim to circumvent them cannot be resolved without the intervention of a mediating operation of validation that can make it possible, on an ongoing basis, to assess the degree of adequacy between the observable and the observed... And we know well that this adequacy can only be outlined on a horizon that is probably infinite, as Jean Ladrière taught us (Piaser and Ladrière 1976). In this process, in which gains and losses are totted up in the search for knowledge, factors outside the research processes themselves also intervene to which it is important to pay attention – for example, in the case we shall outline, we observe a reconfiguration of the general population itself that constitutes here the empirical referential in relation to which our results may be validated.

Before we proceed, we need to better frame this study.

Hidden populations and national surveys of drug use in the general population

Let us start from one of the definitions of hidden populations that can be given: "a subset of the general population whose membership is not readily distinguished or enumerated based on existing knowledge and/or sampling capabilities" (Wiebel 1990, quoted in Fitzgerald 1996, 7). D. Heckathorn (1997) gets closer to the substance of these populations when, in addition to the impossibility of aligning them with a survey framework, he includes in the definition the facts that serious concerns are involved with the privacy of their behaviours and that they are associated with stigmatised or illegal activities, suggesting that any accounts that are made of them are unreliable.

In fact, when a survey is conducted in the general population to measure the prevalence of drug use, there are few previously known characteristics of the target populations that allow for any sample design. As a result, and paradoxically, a sample used in a survey on drug use among general population is defined precisely in a negative way: it is a sample that is not built up on the basis of the relationship of the populations with consumption — which is precisely the characteristic that is intended to be known.

There is a completely opposite situation in surveys aimed at studying the behaviour and characteristics of "problem drug users": in this case, individuals known to institutions are targeted precisely because they consume and because this consumption causes them problems. Also contrasting with the methodology of general population surveys are approaches that select the survey population by means of the "snowball" technique. In these cases, it is a question of starting from known consumption situations and users in order to reach people who share similar characteristics.

The survey among general population thus excludes the possibility of selecting the target population by taking into account the characteristics of the populations whose behaviour we want to know. What then is the justification for this type of survey, if the number of drug users with problems can, in general, be accurately known through the records of institutions and if samples built through the "snowball" technique are usually considered as "particularly useful for located hidden populations" (Morgan 2008)? Moreover, these samples, which are often small in size, also offer the advantage of allowing a deeper understanding of individual behaviours. We would like to cite two reasons for opting to survey the general population: one of a political and the other of a scientific nature.

At the political level, the request for surveys of the general population is framed by a concern for knowledge that can directly serve the management of the social problem represented by the drug use and which is linked to a high degree of social urgency. Considering prevention or treatment relative to this function of management, the ideal for the manager would be to have direct indicators allowing him to identify, as far as possible in real time, the nature and extent of the problems. It happened that one of these managers of risk behaviours presents his needs to the research team, suggesting that he should be provided with a "control panel" such as pilots have, with flashing lights, allowing him perfect control of situations. This "control panel" metaphor was, historically, at the origin and development of studies of "social indicators" in the United States, essentially in the 1950s and 60s — an experience to which we will return in Chapter 1.

In the particular case of surveys of the general population focussing on behaviours related to the drugs use, the first studies were conducted in 1979 in the United States and Canada, after an initial period of studies dedicated to populations considered to be at risk (young people, prisoners...).

Following the experience in the United States, the concern with the centralised management of problems in a large, multinational space such as the European Union motivated a new temporality in the methodology of social indicators. These indicators are considered to be all the better if they are part of sets or batteries of indicators that are consensual, general and capable of formatting the definition of the problems that are being targeted.

It was with this end in view that "observatories" were set up, backed up at national level by "focal points" to process information, and a European Monitoring Centre for Drugs and Drug Addiction (EMCDDA) established, taking over some of the concerns of the Pompidou Group that had functioned before, and continued to function, within the Council of Europe.

The concern here is to achieve the most complete standardisation possible of guidelines and tools for collecting information. Our research practice in the area of consumption took root within the Pompidou Group and we have been part, since its creation, of the EMCDDA's expert group on General Population Surveys (GPS). In addition, the questionnaire we use to measure consumption includes batteries of questions proposed by the EMCDDA as "models" to be replicated in the various national studies.

While it is easy to understand the motivations behind this type of approach, it is not difficult to understand some of the risks involved. We should like to highlight two of them, with the first relating to the application on an international scale of batteries of indicators constructed with reference to a problem defined at the intersection of many national realities (the reasoning does not change if we say that these indicators may be inspired by the research traditions of countries with a longer track record in the area) may impose an understanding of the problems on "large spaces", neglecting the possibilities of an understanding that is more rooted in medium-sized or small territories. This difficulty is due to factors of two orders: on the one hand, the fact that surveys are expensive and do not allow levels of representativity of smaller spaces. and on the other, the need to reach a consensus at international level to define the indicators does not allow the cultural specificities of regions or even countries to be taken into account. This uprooting of indicators from local realities makes it easier progressively to strengthen the epidemiological orientation of the studies.

The solution that makes it possible to benefit from the international dimension while at the same time valuing the national anchoring of the problem of consumption may be to complement epidemiological indicators, which mainly express quantities, with knowledge of the meaning of behaviours that can be obtained, for example, by sociology. We must admit that it has not been easy to achieve this desirable complementarity, given on the one hand the limits on the length of questionnaires and, on the other, the dominance in the context of our type of study of the epidemiological point of view, reinforced by the reduction of the number of behaviours to be "monitored", due to the broadening of potentially addictive behaviours.

We thus arrive at a situation that is somewhat paradoxical, and this is the second risk that we wished to highlight: the agreed effort to bring to light the risk behaviours of a hidden population may end up concealing important dimensions of these behaviours. The masking of these dimensions, albeit undoubtedly justified by the need to clarify others, and not specific to this area nor to this type of surveys, is all the more likely to occur as the indicators measured by the observation instruments are, as we have said, standardised and have a universal vocation — to serve the purposes of international comparison. It is also the case that the knowledge thus obtained tends to be imposed as the only kind available on the problems in question, insofar as these surveys cannot easily be carried out beyond large public institutions, due to the costs involved.

The social sciences are accustomed to managing this type of paradox. We thus come to the second order of reasons—those of a scientific nature—that can motivate the conducting of surveys on the general population.

In another paper (Balsa 2020b) we analysed the ways in which the social sciences and the political and administrative sciences have been involved in the implementation of public policy in the United States over the last century. Indeed, the development of studies on social indicators, as mentioned earlier, was important in driving the development of sociology in the United States, especially its quantitative aspect. The same type of interest is undoubtedly present in the particular case of surveys on the drug use in the general population. Works of this nature are extremely stimulating for researchers, insofar as they see themselves directly involved in the construction of a pressing social problem that involves actors of different natures (in terms of disciplinary area or institutions of origin, or even in terms of different levels of involvement in the problems) and who therefore act in different areas of legitimacy. Then, due to the nature of the subject, the challenge posed to research in accounting for behaviours that tend to be hidden and to define hidden populations sharply challenges the methodology and requires a sharpening of technical ingenuity. These are the challenges that motivate the production of this book. We want to share and at the same time open up a space for debate on the definition of epistemological stances, theorising approaches, strategies and instruments capable of highlighting the possible responses to these challenges.

In the next three chapters we shall try to report on the strategies we adopted to analyse consumption behaviours that, given the normative contexts in which they take place, are hidden. We pay most attention, of course, to our experience in conducting the survey on the use of psychoactive substances in the resident population in Portugal. For this, we will summarise the distinction we made earlier between opacity and dissimulation. The opacity, we stated, has to do with the contingencies inherent to the researcher and the research instruments. Regardless of the opacity presented by behaviours—and we know that they are always complex—it interests us here to consider, given that this is an effort to reflect on methodology, the modalities through which research produces knowledge, by successive approximations and no doubt always in a partial manner. Dissimulation, on the contrary, is a prerogative that belongs entirely to individuals, when questioned about their practices or the meanings they give to them. In certain circumstances, they may have sufficient reasons to conceal practices or meanings, or to reveal them only partially, or to declare practices or meanings that do not correspond to the experiences they hold to be true.

Finally, when it is a question, as in our case, of studying the evolution of these behaviours over time, it may happen that the instruments we use to validate and control the answers, in an attempt to circumvent opacity and dissimulation, reveal to us that the "truth" of consumption may hide behind an insidious and not immediately perceptible change in the structure of the target population of the study — the resident population of Portugal. We shall detail this analysis in the third chapter. Before that, in the first chapter, we shall discuss opacity and then, in the second, dissimulation.

CHAPTER 1

OPACITY:
METHODOLOGICAL CHALLENGES OF SURVEYS ON DRUG USE IN THE GENERAL POPULATION

The tradition of general population surveys, in the case of drug use in particular, has been studied in the literature, in its different technical and scientific dimensions (EMCDDA 2002; Beck 2006; Abraham et al. 1999). We will leave the discussion of some of these dimensions for later, when we present our questionnaire. For now, we should like to focus on some questions that the use of this information gathering technique may pose from a methodological point of view.

The review of literature that, with this same objective, has been undertaken by Timothy Johnson lists the main dimensions of what are considered "sources of error" of "general population surveys" on the prevalence of substance use, despite the high quality that is recognised in some of its applications (Johnson 2014). Given that this work has already been done, we are here more interested in considering these "sources of error" based on our own experience, which is what we propose to reflect upon here.

Based on Paul J. Lavrakas's (2013) reworking of the "total survey error" model, Johnson develops a systematisation around two categories: 1) "representation errors" and 2) "measurement errors". Representation errors arise from technical problems that prevent the survey from correctly representing the population to which it is applied, and include operations associated with: a) the coverage of the target population; b) the operationalisation of the sample design; c) the exhaustiveness of the collection of information, in terms both of the individuals selected and of the questions in the questionnaire; and d) the weighting of results. Measurement errors, in turn, call into question the survey's ability to adequately measure the objects it aims to apprehend, and may arise from: a) the operationalisation of concepts in indicators; b) the formulation or organisation of the questions, when they do not allow of a correct approximation to the objects; c) the processing and analysis of the data; and d) the interpretation of or causal inferences made on the basis of the results.

This type of approach raises some questions insofar as, on the one hand, it is inspired by a moral conception of error (presuming that it would be possible, through "good" methodological practice, to know the "truth" of an object represented as being totally transparent) and, on the other hand, is limited to operations directly controlled by the researchers, so neglecting the interventions of other significant actors that are also associated with the construction of the surveys. This limitation cannot be justified by a desire to achieve more precise measurements, since not even the very measurement "errors" attributed to the researchers are differentiated in the calculations, since the whole set of "errors" is represented by a single coefficient.

The idea of error, as it is developed, is based on positivist reasoning according to which reality is transparent and total knowledge of it is possible, dependent only on the quality of the measuring instruments used. By contrast, we think that the process of scientific production cannot be represented based on these assumptions. This is because knowledge about censored behaviours, as probably with any other kind of behaviours, is not transparent; at the same time, as we shall seek to demonstrate below, the behaviours are not only not transparent, but deliberately concealed. For this reason, we cannot expect that the suggested project of arriving at knowledge of a reality depends only on the efforts that the researcher would make in order not to commit errors (which is not to say that the researcher cannot make mistakes and that he should not try to avoid them). In this sense, the most reasonable thing to do is to start from the principle that the research process aims to bring knowledge as close as possible to reality; however, from this approximation will result a remainder that will always remain unknown, because knowledge is dynamic and delimited by a probably irresolvable tension between an observable and what we can actually observe (cf. Ladrière 1976).

It is in this sense that the bid to attain knowledge cannot be achieved only with the competence of the researcher and the excellence of their research instruments; on the contrary, it depends on many other factors, which may be material, human or social. Even limiting ourselves to the logic of scientific production itself and specifically to the construction of surveys on the general population, the instruments and guidelines adopted always depend, at the very least, on political and normative benchmarks that may constrain their results — as we shall try to show below.

For these reasons, we shall integrate the abovementioned “sources of error” in a schema that is more compatible with the possibility of including the responsibility of the researcher, which can neither be negotiated nor delegated, in a wider set of operations involving a larger number of actors; thus, we shall take into account:

A. **Political and normative referentials of survey construction**
   a) Disciplines and problematics of the survey as instruments of knowledge and opacity
   b) Survey as instrument of a political referential that imposes on it a way of looking
B. **Construction of survey populations**
   a) Sample design
   b) Construction of field sample
   c) Weighting operations (correction of the sample taken)
C. **Construction of the questionnaire**
   a) Operationalisation of the concepts or theoretical frameworks
   b) Questionnaire size
   c) Formulation of questions
   d) Definition of measurement criteria
   e) Definition of filters
D. **Technical conditions of fieldwork aimed at increasing the quality of the information gathered**
   a) Avoiding the alarm effect
   b) Ensuring credibility of teams involved in conducting the survey
   c) Conditions under which questionnaire is administered
   d) Quality of controls, at different levels
E. **Information gathered in both theoretical and realised samples, and what it means**
   a) Construction of sample actually realized
   b) Non-response at levels of selected households and individuals
   c) Non-responses to specific questions in questionnaire
   d) Weightings

F. Quality of interpretation and generalisation of results

a) Processing errors
b) Inference errors

This is the grid of difficulties of general population surveys on drugs use that we shall develop below.

Political and normative referentials of the survey

In order to analyse a first dimension of the opacity with which the researcher is presented in his objects of study and the ways in which he can integrate this in his work, we shall first focus on the external conditions, from which we shall focus on the political and normative benchmarks related to consumption that condition the research architecture and strategy. We consider the following aspects:

- Disciplines and problematics of the survey as instruments of knowledge and opacity,
- Management of opacity by political benchmarks and by the definition of the social purposes of the survey.

Disciplines and problematics of the survey as instruments of knowledge and opacity

As previously mentioned, the construction of a sample prior to the application of a questionnaire to evaluate the drug use in the general population does not consider, from the outset, any criterion associated with a particular type of consumption, considering as it does only characteristics that ensure the representativeness of the sample (place of residence, gender and age). This is what defines a "general population" — obviously always subject to the age limits that we wish to impose on it. The drug users known to exist within this population constitute, from this point of view, a hidden population, in the sense that it is dissimulated within the vast and varied set of characteristics that may be attributed to this "general population". Strictly speaking, the consumer population hides behind all the characteristics of the population, that is, behind all the singularities that mark each individual's existence and the whole experiential field associated with human activity.

The opacity is, at this level, complete. In fact, we can only overcome this opacity through observation supported by the series of questions in the questionnaire, and this clarification is therefore achieved—in line with the canonical orientations of the methodology—by defining the problematic (linked to some theoretical framework susceptible of engaging an explanatory narrative) of a process of conceptual unravelling and of the formulation of questions that will then be operationalised in the form of variables.

It is thus clear that the construction of the questionnaire is of great importance from the perspective of knowledge about these populations. This is because it is through the questionnaire, in the areas of visibility that are progressively torn open by the questions, by the instructions imposed on their administration and by the filters that condition them, that the opacity associated with hidden behaviours may be overcome — albeit probably always only partially.

We can imagine a questionnaire applied to the entire population that has only one simple question: to find out, for example, whether in their lifetime the individuals surveyed had ever used psychoactive substances. The information obtained in this questionnaire would divide the population into two parts according to the responses collected. The result would lead to the least possible knowledge of the population, indeed reducing it to a Manichean representation that would assume the exclusion of all its other characteristics. With an additional question that would allow us to know, for example, whether individuals who had consumed at some time in their lives were still consuming, we would update our knowledge about the behaviour of the population and could satisfactorily respond to the concerns of a public health manager, who would make decisions according to the value that the prevalence rate might indicate.

This fictitious questionnaire would obviously not enable us to answer the questions that managers of the problem of consumption may themselves ask from the perspective of prevention, for example. But not many more questions are needed to construct the (admittedly minimalist) battery of questions that the EMCDDA proposes as the basis of the model of the European questionnaire, which is based on an epidemiological concern: to delimit risk groups in relation to consumption, taking into account the most important estimated parameters (such as gender, age, type of habitat and region of residence) from the perspective of prevention. As sociologists, and in accordance with the fundamental objectives of an epidemiological reading, we have tried, within the narrow limits imposed by the duration of the application of the questionnaire, to increase the number of intervening variables in order to broaden the possibilities of explanation or understanding of consumption. Thus, in the questionnaires we applied in the first phases of the study, we introduced batteries of questions on sociability, on disruptive situations and on socio-professional status, as a basis for social positioning. No doubt a questionnaire designed by psychologists or economists would prioritise other sets of variables[3].

This differentiation in the perspectives adopted to study drug use can also be seen when we consider all national surveys on the subject. In some questionnaires the predominant issue is health (France and Denmark) or mental health (Greece); in others, crime-related issues dominate (United Kingdom); in still others, drug use is one of the topics considered in cross-thematic questionnaires (Sweden and Ireland). According to François Beck (Beck 2006, 69), from the end of the 1990s health and risk management issues tend to predominate.

Portugal's questionnaire began within a framework of the problematic of social networks and sociabilities. However, this orientation was gradually abandoned in order to respond to the extension of public health concerns to other types of non-substance dependence (such as gambling and the internet) and to the need to deepen the knowledge of others (such as alcohol or new substances). In another chapter we shall present our options in more detail, as well as the circumstances that underpinned these changes.

Each questionnaire is thus constructed based on a representation that the researcher makes of the population, taking into account the problem that is being studied. The representation of the target population underlying the model questionnaire suggested by the EMCDDA is an example of a representation of consumption centred on an epidemiological perspective,

---

[3] We have analysed, in the context of national surveys on the prevention of HIV/AIDS, how different disciplinary areas of the promoters of the studies led to very different problematisations and the choice of variables (Casimiro Balsa, *La Constitution d'une banque d'indicateurs: vers une approche comparative internationale dans le domaine des comportements sexuels et des attitudes face au risque HIV*, Facultés Saint-Louis, Bruxelles, 32 pp.). See also the doctoral thesis of François Beck (Beck 2006).

with consumption stripped of much of its sociological context. This is consumption without a consumer or where the consumer is all but reduced to morphological dimensions: gender, age and place of residence.

It is the case, however, that behind each consumption there is not just a man or a woman or a certain age group but a social individual, socio-professional itinerary and situation; a school experience, a training pathway, a status and a certain array of family rhythms and codes; an area where other sociabilities take place in which more or fewer friends feature, as well as confidants, accomplices in adventures or maybe just companions in boredom; habitual spaces and places, and a number of routines. When we consider consumption stripped of its context, it is this density that is hidden. When, in addition to consumption, we consider the person who engages in it, we realise that it is in this universe, which constitutes the daily life of each one of us, that the vast majority of drug users are hidden. It is this density and this daily life that explain the opacity that the object of consumption presents to the researcher, and which mobilise his instruments of observation. A large proportion of drug users are, for the most part, embedded in banal scenarios. The image of the consumer who is completely wrapped up in his consumption, who unfortunately exists, cannot replace the representation of ordinary consumption.

This is why we have some difficulty in distinguishing the sociological profiles of drug users from those of the rest of the population... in general! Moreover, in the vast majority of cases, the first consumption of a substance, like any subsequent consumption, does not require any break in the habitual routines of those who consume, and the suppliers of the substance are generally people who are familiar or close to the consumer[4].

Setting aside the minority of drug users whose consumption is problematic (a phenomenon whose seriousness we do not want to question), the majority can be found within a regular framework of daily life and conventional normative contexts.

Of course, beyond the opacity effect it implies, their being embedded in these contexts still raises the question of the dissimulation of behaviours, in cases where there is a clear skewing of these normative frameworks. This

---

[4] These questions will be developed in a paper devoted specifically to the analysis of consumption and consuming populations.

involves the issue of normative diffraction (cf. Balsa 2019), which we will analyse in the next chapter.

This margin for manoeuvre that the researcher has in proceeding with the characterisation of the contexts and circumstances of consumption marks the difference between the epidemiological reason and the sociological reason present in the construction of all questionnaires. Behind each collection protocol there is always a mode of construction of the subject of consumption. Each of these constructions reveals and at the same time hides all the conditions and circumstances that may contribute to the consumption having a meaning for the consumer.

Management of opacity by political referentials and by the definition of the social purposes of the survey

In the same way that the questionnaire is an instrument of a theory, when the objective is the validation of theoretical frameworks, it is also an instrument that serves a social purpose, from the point of view of oriented research — that is, in the cases where, as in our discussion, it is conducted in a dynamic of support for political decision-making. Of course, the boundary between the two purposes is not always rigid, nor clear, and its management will depend very much on experience, on the research tradition and on the flexibility left to the research teams. We saw earlier how, in this sense, consumer studies in Europe are framed by different problems depending on the country. It is also reasonable to think that the scientific capital previously accumulated by a research team should be invested in the construction of a narrative adapted to the problem to be solved.

However, due to the status of the study as an instrument to support decision-making, it is understandable that political-administrative bodies should play an important role in defining the areas of opacity of the objects it wishes to see clarified, especially in cases where the initiative and funding (generally significant) of the work programmes come from them.

This definition by political-administrative bodies of the research subjects to be prioritised may be subordinated to national or transnational political referentials (Muller 2000), as in the case of the guidelines promoted by the EMCDDA. In both cases, these benchmarks change as the problems are reformulated. In the case of Portugal, with which we are concerned, the benchmark that determined the organisation of the first application of the study, in 2001, was initially indexed to a situation of social alarm relating to drug use and later to the start of the policy of decriminalisation of consumption. This representation of the problem allowed an opening, both for the epidemiological approach and for the knowledge of the circumstances likely to be associated with consumption. Gradually, as knowledge about the consumption of illicit substances was established, attention was also directed towards the consumption of alcohol, interest in which was more sustained than that in the consumption of tobacco (a theme that came more to the fore during the public debate on the prohibition of smoking in public places). The focus then switched to gambling for money and internet dependence, based on the development of the problematic of non-substance dependence.

The increasing diversity of foci around which the problems were reformulated left ever less space in the questionnaire for questions more motivated by the theoretical problematics mentioned above, so imposing the epidemiological on the sociological perspective.

Regardless of any assessment that may be made on how these reformulations contribute to the clarification of the problems or to the definition of ways to solve them, it is a fact that political referentials and the definition of the social purposes of the research contribute, to an important extent, to densifying or, on the contrary, to attenuating the opacity with which the objects of study always present themselves to research.

Construction of survey populations

We may also consider, in conjunction with the administration of the questionnaire, that the opacity of drug use may be reduced in the phases of the study in which the reference universe of the study is decided (to find out about certain types of use, the lower and upper limits of the reference populations are not identical) and the sampling plan and the rules allowing the construction of the sample in the field are defined.
This construction then involves the following operations:

- design of the sampling plan (theoretical sample),
- construction of the sample in the field (realised sample),

- weighting operations (adjustment of realised sample to theoretical sample).

These themes will be developed in the fourth part of this work, as they require too much technical development for our argument in this chapter.

Construction of the questionnaire

After the definition of the survey population, the construction of the questionnaire is an important node around which much of the constant tension is played out that the researcher must manage between the unveiling of and the opacity of the facts. We have already referred in the Introduction to the dimensions and consequences that these questions have on the political referentials that condition the study. We shall now approach them from a more methodological point of view.

Operationalisation of theoretical concepts or frameworks

As this is essentially a survey aimed at collecting information to support decision-making within the scope of public policies, the formulation of some of the questions is motivated more by the priorities assigned to the social problems involved and their dimensions than by the need to validate theoretical frameworks defined *a priori*. It is clear that questions are not assembled without formulating narratives about the motivations or circumstances of behaviours. These narratives are sometimes based on results that have become sedimented in the specialist literature. In some cases, especially when disciplinary issues may come to the fore, questions serve theoretical rationales that tend to build an explanatory framework for the behaviours: the introduction of questions about sociability or disruptive situations, for example, is due to theoretical postulates whose validation is sought. This pragmatism in the construction of the questionnaire does not, however, prevent all the materials collected constituting starting points for theoretical constructions *a posteriori*. Fundamentally, this is what we seek to do in undertakings such as this one that seek to better frame the results that we present in more technical reports.

Formulation of questions

In general, the themes addressed in the questionnaires take into account, on the one hand, changes in consumption behaviours and, on the other, the progressive extension of markets to new substances, the redefinition of the social use of the old ones and political sensitivity to new forms of dependence. The contemporary definition of the drug problem will thus be dominated by three factors: the democratisation of consumption, the redefinition of the social uses of drugs, and the reformulation of the regulatory and legal frameworks linked to consumption. These trends will be translated in the design of questionnaires aimed at the general population and, in some cases, motivate in-depth investigations of some populations or particular themes.

Many of the questions, especially those related to prevalence and circumstances of use, are formatted according to international standards as part of the transnational comparison programme conducted by the European Monitoring Centre for Drugs and Drug Addiction. Other questions are codified within the framework of different scales of measurement of consumption or its consequences, which are also shared by different international studies. In these cases, the difficulty may present itself in terms of the adaptation of the parameters used to the experiences of each country or even of each context in which the questionnaire is applied. We can say that, in cases where local sensitivities are respected less, the hope is that this loss is compensated by the gain obtained in terms of the comparison of information at the level of large spaces.

Questionnaire size

For the reasons already mentioned, the extension of the survey to new substances, the agreed political priority given to others, and the importance assumed by non-substance dependencies have increased the length of our questionnaire, even though we have eliminated questions that allowed a better sociological contextualisation of consumption. Proving once and for all the unverifiable assertion of manuals of methodology, according to which questionnaires are always too long, ours really is long. The average application time is 45 minutes.

However, it is a structured questionnaire based on multiple consumer profiles and the multiple positions they can assume, which means that the people interviewed are not confronted with all the questions. This does not mean that its application does not require competent interviewers and careful preparation in order to lessen the difficulty it presents and to reduce fatigue and its effects on the quality of the information. We shall detail below how we do this.

Definition of criteria of measurement

It is not of interest to us here to discuss "measurement" in the sense in which operationalists of the positivist tradition understand it, requiring that each indicator used has a correspondent at the conceptual level and for each concept to fit into a perfectly codified theory. This position of ours is justified by the considerations made earlier, even if they should not be interpreted as some form of disrespect with regard to the rigour with which the formulation of thc qucstions should be treated; however, their relevance applies in all cases, and not only in the particular modality of the survey of the general population that we are interested in discussing here.

However, measurement takes on an important connotation for us when we consider the "measurement" of the behaviours we wish to observe or the measurement of the consequences that these behaviours may have. The entire political and institutional framework of the survey is focused on this purpose of the study, and this justifies the efforts at harmonisation to which we have already referred.

This does not mean, however, that the measurements may not make sense or correspond to possible expectations in relation to certain experiences. Successive consensual efforts to construct, update, validate or compare different measures with each other confirm that measurement should be subject to a continuous approach, rather than aiming to fix it at any one time, once and for all (Peretti-Watel, Beck and Legleye 2007; Legleye et al. 2013; Legleye 2018; Legleye et al. 2015).

The greater sensitivity of tests to certain populations also justifies the simultaneous use of different measures. In our survey we have been applying appropriate tests to the various substances, with the possibility of applying different tests to the same substance: the American Psychiatric

Association's DSM (Diagnostic and Statistical Manual of Mental Disorders), for various substances; the AUDIT (Alcohol Use Disorders Identification Test), developed by the World Health Organization, and the CAGE[5] questionnaire for problem drinking and potential alcohol problems; the CAST (Cannabis Abuse Screening Test) and the SDS (Severity of Dependence Scale), for cannabis; and the Fagerström Test, for tobacco.

A discussion of the difficulties that measurement can pose in the particular case of alcohol use is presented in part 3.

Definition of filters

As this is an instrument aimed at observing the use of multiple substances and intended for populations with very different consumption profiles, the survey for the general population is structured based on a system of filters. The application of the questionnaire through the CAPI (computer-assisted personal interviewing) technique facilitates the management of these filters.

Use of show cards

In the case of questions that require a more laborious positioning, the use of show cards detailing all the response modalities is another tool we use to support the interviewee and to avoid inaccuracies or errors in the answers.

The use of show cards also means that substances are not verbalised during the interview relationship, thus reinforcing the confidentiality of statements in cases where someone else may be nearby.

Technical conditions of fieldwork aimed at improving quality of information collected

As we shall see in the following chapter, dissimulation insinuates itself into consumer relations in a very decisive way, although through strategies that may differ greatly. For this reason, the application of the questionnaire has to be thought through with particular care, in order to lessen possible

[5] The acronym "CAGE" is related to the questions on Cutting down, Annoyance by criticism, Guilty feeling, and Eye-openers.

resistance to an enquiry about a dimension that definitely belongs to an area of intimacy for individuals.

The question we asked ourselves was under what circumstances an individual would be willing to respond when someone he does not know knocks on his door to ask if he uses drugs.

The preparation for the application of the questionnaire in the field is thus preceded by a set of operations that we list below.

Avoiding the alarm effect

When first building the sample, distributed across a set of randomly selected statistical sub-sections in all the municipalities of the country (see Part IV), we set the number of interviews to be conducted at each sampling point in order to avoid the alarm effect. This effect could occur if, for example, in a given population cluster—generally small in size—the entire population were selected. For this reason, the average number of interviews per sample point was set at 10, and could range between 7 and 12, according to the population density of the sub-section. Since the sample is by area, each conglomerate selected at random constitutes its centre, and it is possible in cases where the sub-section has a very small population to cluster lodgings from a neighbouring sub-section in order to distribute the lodgings to be selected in a spaced (and equally random) manner.

Ensuring credibility of teams associated with information gathering

One of the conditions put forward by the participants in a qualitative study that we conducted, precisely in terms of preparation of fieldwork (cf. analysis of this study in the following chapter), was the credibility that they were able to associate with the institution and the survey team members who presented themselves to apply the questionnaire.

Since this was known, any contact made by the team carrying out fieldwork at the selected accommodation was preceded by the sending of a letter on the part of the university institution carrying out the study, signed by the researcher in charge.

This letter presented the commissioning authority, in this case SICAD (General Directorate for Intervention on Addictive Behaviours and

Dependencies), and the main objectives of the study, stressing the need for knowledge about certain behaviours from a public health perspective. It also stated that the selection of the accommodation was made in a fully randomised way. The postal address of the institution responsible for the study and the company carrying out the fieldwork were also given. The letter also provided the central telephone number of the university institution so that someone from the selected accommodation could confirm the information provided or clarify any questions related to the application. Any such call was forwarded to a member of the research team.

Conditions of questionnaire administration

Since the interview was conducted in the homes of the selected individuals, the application was prepared so as to guarantee maximum confidentiality of the responses provided. It is indeed difficult to expect an interviewee to provide reliable information when, as one of the interviewees told us during a preparatory phase of the study, "you have your whole family leaning over you...".

To overcome this difficulty, the application is carried out employing the CAPI (computer-assisted personal interviewing) technique, which ensures that the questions are not visible to any of the possible participants. As a matter of principle, moreover, the interview should be conducted out without the presence of third parties. In practice, this happens in the vast majority of cases: in the application of the study in 2016/17, in 93% of cases the interview was conducted with only the interviewee present.

In the same way, no substance is mentioned in the wording of the question. This information is transmitted to the interviewee via cards, with the result that the respondent does not have to verbalise the name of the substance in order to respond.

Validation of responses through checks on verisimilitude, internal consistency and degree of confidence merited from interviewer's point of view

As with other questionnaires, this one also registers the degree of confidence that the responses merit from the point of view of the interviewer. Based on the application of the Survey in 2016/17, in the vast majority of cases

(77.4%) confidence in the information provided is "very high" or "high"; if we add to this the "sufficient" degree of confidence, the information collected is considered reliable in 98.7% of interviews.

At another level, during fieldwork, an analysis of the internal consistency of the responses is regularly undertaken. This procedure enables the detection of inconsistencies between responses and, if justified, the cancellation of the questionnaires concerned.

The validity of responses is also checked in the sense of their plausibility, either concerning the whole territory or certain regions, or on certain response guidelines which do not comply with the principle of fidelity due to any longitudinal application.

These checks are aimed not only at verifying inconsistencies in interviewees' statements but also, through these, possible problems related to the information gathering itself.

In chapter 3 of this section, we present an analysis of the validity of guidelines for results that did not meet expectations, considering knowledge of the population's positions that was obtained in previous applications. This analysis does, in fact, allow us to introduce a factor—the change in population structure—that may disturb the principle of fidelity of the results obtained and which has nothing to do with the quality of the information provided or of the collection instruments or procedures.

Since this is a nationally representative sample, we can also indirectly validate the quality of coverage of the target population by examining how the data collected respects the distributions of its characteristics, measured through the census conducted by the INE (National Statistics Institute), considering the age categories we are interested in (ages 15-74). In addition to the characteristics that served to construct the sample—gender, age and place of residence—we can also carry out checks using other characteristics that should also be represented in our sample in the proportion they account for in the national population (e.g. marital status, levels of education, etc.).

Information gathered for theoretical and realised sample: non-responses as first sign of concealment?

When analysing the results of a questionnaire several categories, which are often not interpreted or are misinterpreted—"non-response", "don't know" and "refuses to answer"—signify positions of concealment. As we will see in the next chapter, concealment can take different modalities. In addition to direct concealment, to which the different forms of absence of information may correspond, we may also consider those resulting from the relationship of trust/distrust that insinuates itself in an interview. André Petitat thus distinguishes[6]: the "lie", when an occurrence is illegitimately transformed (from the perspective of the prevailing codes of communication); the "unsaid", when something is illegitimately concealed by omission; and the "intimacy or discretion", when the omission may be considered legitimate, as far as occurrences considered to be in the field of people's intimacy are concerned.

These various categories will be analysed in more detail in the next chapter. Limiting ourselves here to the restrictions on access to information that may occur in the application phase of the questionnaire, we will consider: 1) the construction of the sample actually carried out; 2) non-response at the levels of the selected household and individual; and 3) the quality of the information provided.

Construction of the actually realised sample

The response rates obtained have to be seen with reference to the culture of the surveying contexts and may vary from country to country (EMCDDA 2002, 82); they may also vary with the collection technique used, as we shall show in another chapter. In our case we employed face-to-face interviews, using the CAPI (computer-assisted personal interviewing) collection technique.

It is clear that the conditions imposed for the selection of the information units (households contacted) and of the individual respondents within the household may facilitate more or less the obtention of information. In our case we tried to follow a strict protocol, as already explained, given the objective of ensuring that the sample was as representative as possible of

[6] This axis is constructed on the basis of three vectors that structure an actor's relationship with others: "visibility" (to show or hide oneself), "metamorphosis" (to deform or authentically transmit one's experience) and "normativity" (to respect or transgress the rules of communication) (A Petitat, "Secret et morphogenèse sociale" manuscript, undated, Lausanne, 20 pp.).

the general population, despite not having survey bases at national level for the whole population.

Having guaranteed the quality of the theoretical sample, our next concern is to ensure that its implementation in the field does not introduce any biases that may distort it. With this in view, we seek to eliminate as far as possible the intervention of members of the team responsible for the fieldwork during the phase of selecting respondents. This phase includes the mapping and subsequent selection of households within the previously defined survey units (statistical sub-sections), and the selection of the respondent within the household.

In this process, the most important principle is that which excludes any possibility of substitution by field workers of the randomly selected units. The need for such substitutions may occur in various situations. At the household selection level, it can happen that the selected unit does not correspond to a family residence, that the house is not inhabited or that the resident is absent for a long period of time[7]. In these cases, the field team has a list of substitute accommodation, compiled according to the same criteria as the first one, from which the non-viable accommodation can be replaced. Another situation is where the home can be contacted but refuses to respond. In this case the principle of non-substitution applies. Substitution is also not allowed when one can move on to selecting the individual within the household, and the interview is made non-viable by a refusal or the systematic absence of the selected individual.

In the course of the different applications of the study, two strategies have been followed in the face of these types of "non-response". Initially, we chose to follow the principle of non-substitution in a strict manner, that is, the programmed sample could not be carried out. In 2001, for example, of the projected sample of 15,000 individuals only 14,184 interviews were conducted. Later on, however, we chose to replace these cases, but following a set of conditions that we shall explain below.

The principle of non-substitution obviously tends to safeguard the randomness of the sample, as well as the type and quality of representativeness thus obtained; we know that not observing it alters the results obtained,

[7] The last two situations require confirmation from neighbours.

namely in terms of the number of declarations of consumption recorded. Two results allow us to demonstrate this relationship.

In a first step, we conducted a test, limited to densely populated urban areas, to assess the possible distortion effect introduced into the results with a selection of individuals in which those households and individuals that could not be contacted according to the defined rules were allowed to be substituted. These substitutions could be made following, this time, the random route technique.

In the following tables we present the results of the comparison. Regardless of the size of the difference, which must be viewed with some caution[8], the orientation is clear in the sense that the selection rules contribute to produce the representation of the consumer subject. In fact, whatever the prevalence indicator considered (lifetime, last year and last month), consumption statements are always higher when substitution has been allowed.

Table 1-1. Prevalence of lifetime use, last 12 months and last 30 days in two types of sample: with and without substitutions

	Lifetime prevalences		**Last 12 months prevalences**		**Last 30 days prevalences**	
	Sample A (INPG)*	*Sample B* (INPG)*	*Sample A* (INPG)*	*Sample B* (INPG)*	*Sample A* (INPG)*	*Sample B* (INPG)*
Cannabis	8.6	12.9	2.8	6	2.6	4.3
Ecstasy	1.8	1.4	1.1	1.1	0.2	0.5
Amphetamines	0.4	2.2	0.4	1.1	-	0.6
Cocaine	2.5	4.5	1.2	2.6	0.7	1.3
Heroin	1.3	1.6	0.6	0.9	0.3	0.2
LSD	0.2	0.6	0.2	0.6	-	0.3

* Sample A: without replacements; Sample B: with replacements

How can this result be interpreted? Different variables have to be equated. We shall do so according to the following model:

---

[8] The differences found should be interpreted with some caution, since due to the limited number of individuals who participated in the test, the margins of error are considerable.

- We agree that what we are interested in explaining is the orientation of the consumption statement (yes or no) and we shall use the other variables as having the potential to be explanatory;
- We are particularly interested in taking into account the mode of selection adopted, which may vary between allowing and not allowing the individual to be substituted;
- Then, if substitution is allowed, the question arises as to which criterion is to be adopted. Two possibilities were considered: substitution, based on a certain profile of individual, or substitution on a random basis;
- Finally, we consider that the reading of the results can be made based on two different hypotheses: in one case we accept that individuals tend, at the outset, to hide consumption; the opposite hypothesis assumes that the communication of results is transparent.

Let us then make a first reading that explains the results obtained: in substitution mode, the number of declarations of consumption increases. This occurs because there is no propensity for drug users to hide their behaviour. Therefore, by increasing the population contacted, we increase the probability of finding drug users. On the contrary, by not replacing it, we lose that opportunity. One question remains to be answered: how did the interviewer carry out the substitution? In the test conducted, he chose according to the quotas that needed to be filled. We can conclude that, even if these criteria did not include considerations about the possible consumption habits of the individuals to be met, there was at least a biased choice, that is, a non-random one.

It should be noted that, given the hypothesis that individuals have no propensity to hide their consumption, as considered above, it is indifferent, from the strict perspective of the orientation of the information obtained[9], whether we opt for the substitution or non-substitution method: in these cases, the first selected individual who refused to answer can, in principle, be replaced without consequences by any other individual, as long as the selection criterion does not contain gross biases.

---

[9] Of course, the option is not at all indifferent from the point of view of the status of the sample that will be constructed.

The situation is different when we hypothesise that individuals have some propensity to hide. In this case, and assuming substitutions, the criterion used to make them becomes particularly important, since any individual contacted next will also refuse, for the same reason and so on, until a non-consumer appears and responds. This makes it less likely to register drug users. This is not what happened in the test. So, this result can be explained in two ways: either individuals do not show any propensity to hide (see hypothesis above) or the choice was biased towards finding drug users.

Based on another piece of information we collected, and which will be analysed in the following chapter, we have reasons to start from the hypothesis that drug users have a propensity to hide. Although exceptions are observed, the literature also allows us to confirm this orientation (Johnson 2014, 2-3). Thus, while not fully controlling the selection criteria that field workers may use when they are free to select, we prefer to impose a collection method that does not allow for substitutions.

However, if we consider as above that in some cases substitution is necessary to achieve the theoretical sample as defined, then we must conclude that this can only be carried out within a single random run, with this possibility already provided for at the outset. This is the guideline that we follow, so taking away from field workers any autonomy to make selections outside the list of pre-selected individuals and obliging them to follow the imposed selection rules.

In order to ensure the homogeneity of the answers obtained with and without substitution, we constituted two distinct bases, so that we could control any possible bias.

In this discussion, it is clear that the choices made by the researcher allow us to construct the target population of the study and, in this way, influence the results. This prerogative will become even clearer when, in the second part, we analyse the effects of the survey techniques on the results obtained. This is also the case when, as mentioned earlier, the survey variables are selected, allowing us to show or, on the contrary, to hide certain characteristics of individuals.

For now we would like to conclude on two levels: on the one hand, underscoring the difficulty inherent in comparison exercises, namely those to which we contributed and which are carried out within the EMCDDA, in which studies conducted using a wide variety of techniques and methodologies form a part; at another level, we underscore our choice of more rigorous techniques, where control of the procedures can be done at each step, because only this possibility of control justifies the considerable costs that must be invested to construct a probabilistic sample and representative results.

Non-responses of household and of individuals

Rates of non-response and bias in results

We can estimate the extent of non-response from Table 1-2, which for the four applications already carried out provides the calculated non-response rates considering different coefficients. In a first approximation and focusing on the results of the last application (2016/17) we can see that of the universe of households selected at the outset (contact attempted), only a portion—86.4%—corresponded to family homes in which contact was possible. Of eligible households, 23.4% rejected the possibility of further contact (refusal at household level). When the interview was authorised and it was possible within the household to select the family member who should be interviewed, 27.6% of individuals refused to answer (refusal at individual level).

The following table provides the reasons for contacts of households that did not result in interviews.

Table 1-2. Rates of response by fhase of contact. Years 2001 to 2016/17

	2001	2007	2012	2016/17
Rates of response taking into account **number of interviews requested**	14,184/21,395*100 **66.3**	12,202/14,826*100 **82.3**	6,817/10,798*100 **63.1**	12,023/16,595*100 **72.4**
Rates of response taking into account **number of contacts established**	14,184/23,491*100 **60.4**	12,202/19,128*100 **63.8**	6,817/14,420*100 **47.3**	12,023/21,663*100 **55.5**
Rates of response taking into account **number of contacts attempted**	14,184/28,127*100 **50.4**	12,202/19,552*100 **62.4**	6,817/16,649*100 **40.9**	12,023/25,076*100 **47.9**

Although they have different meanings, refusals at household and individual levels together add up to 44.5%, if considered in relation to all households that could actually be contacted. On a positive reading, this means that the response rate was 55.5%. Compared to previous applications, in the one conducted in 2016/17, a higher rate was obtained than in 2012, but it was lower than the two conducted in the first decade of the century. This result confirms a trend observed in other studies, at the international level, where a progressive decrease in response rates to this type of survey is noted (Schröder 2016; Beullens et al. 2018; Johnson 2014).

How to evaluate these results? At first reading, undoubtedly with disquiet. However, when we put them into perspective, they can be seen as very acceptable, given the scores usually obtained by this type of survey. In Germany, during the same period as our reference here, the response rate to face-to-face interviews, with random sampling, was around 30% (Schröder 2016). In the particular domain of general population surveys concerning HIV, response rates of 60% are reported in Norway and Sweden, but 30% in the UK and Germany (EMCDDA 2002, 82). Billie Bonevsky and colleagues (Bonevsky et al. 2011), in a more recent review of the literature on general population surveys, consider that a response rate of 70% is considered 'good', but that those obtained in health surveys are generally low — less than 30%. In the particular case of surveys of drug use, the team in charge of the survey of the general population in the Netherlands considered that already at the end of the last century "a non-response rate of 45 percent [50 in Amsterdam] is common for face-to-face interviews performed by Statistics Netherlands" (Abraham et al. 1999, 22). In their own studies on drug use, the response rate obtained was actually 59.9% (ibid., 23).

On a broader level, the importance of non-response rates as a means of ensuring the quality of a representative sample is treated in the literature with guidelines that do not always converge (Groves 2006). In fact, there is no agreement on the minimum percentage that should be obtained so that the representation of the population studied is not distorted. On the one hand, Groves (ibid., 647) cites Babbiee[10] (2007, 262) when, based on a review of social science literature, he suggests that "a response rate of at

[10] Babbie, Earl. 2007. *The Practice of Social Research*. 11th ed. Belmont, CA: Wadsworth.

least 50 percent is considered adequate for analysis and reporting. A rate of 60 percent is good; response of 70 percent is very good." On the other hand, other authors believe that response rates below 70% are insufficient, and that a minimum of 85% is needed to ensure that the results obtained are not biased; this is without considering the fact that seminal theories on the representativeness of samples assume that the theoretical sample would be 100%... Taking from this discussion the idea that different non-response rates may be acceptable, the question arises however at what minimums the biases in the measurements may not be. Another more pragmatic way used by Groves (ibid., 646, 667ff.) to pose the question is whether the advantage of employing probability samples for studying large populations, controlling for margins of error, is not jeopardised by increasing non-response rates.

In fact, the relationship between non-response rates and the level of bias in the results is not linear. On this relationship Groves concludes the following: 1) there is no minimum non-response rate below which bias would occur; 2) when it does occur, bias does not affect all results in the same way. At another level, the author concludes that rather than seeking to lower non-response rates, the researcher should consider 1) the research design followed, insofar as it may reduce the resistance of respondents, and 2) the actual reasons for non-responses.

Regarding the research design, we have been explaining how it is thought out at various levels—from the construction of the questionnaire to the programming of fieldwork, including definition of the sample design—in order to achieve good coverage of the target population and its adherence to the survey. Below, we will detail the types of non-response that we have been recording.

Types of non-responses and non-realised sample

Table 1-3 enables us to find out the reasons that, in the application carried out in 2017, prevented contact with the household and an interview with the selected individual.

In 29% of contacts attempted (25,015) it was not possible to contact the selected households, because they were not family homes (9.2%), or because there was no one aged between 15 and 74 in the household (6.2%), or because it was not possible to communicate with the residents (13.6%).

When contact with the household was possible, in 15.2% of cases the interview could not take place, either because the individuals refused to answer (10.4%) or because the selected person could not be located (4.8%).

When contact could be established and the individual selected, we recorded 6.9% of refusals to answer. This means that explicit refusals to respond represent 17.3% of the total of all attempted contacts — if we add to the refusals on the part of individuals the refusals of the households (10.4%).

Table 1-3. Coverage of theoretical sample and construction of actual sample

	N	%
Total attempted contacts	25,075	100.0
Housing outside sample	3,850	15.4
Outside universe (not eligible)	2,296	9.2
Outside quota	1,554	6.2
No contact due to absence of residents	3,413	13.6
Refusal of household	2,613	10.4
Absence from household of selected person	1,218	4.8
Refusal of individual	1,724	6.9
Language barrier/Sickness	32	0.1
Non-valid interviews	203	0.8
Interviews carried out but not valid	154	0.6
Incomplete interviews	49	0.2
Interviews carried out and validated	12,022	48.0

We also noted a residual number (32) of interviews that could not be conducted due to a language barrier or illness.

Finally, 203 interviews were invalidated following checks or because they were incomplete. These invalidated interviews did not follow the procedures correctly: in 67 cases the imposed random route was not followed, in 62 cases the wrong selection of the individual to be interviewed was made and in 25 cases the wrong selection of the housing was made.

How are these results profiled over time, over a 10-year interval? Looking at the same categories in the application of the survey conducted in 2007, whose sample size was identical to that of 2017—at 12,000 individuals—we find that refusals increase over time: between 2007 and 2017 household refusals increase from 8.5% to 10.4% and individual refusals from 4.9% to 6.9%. By contrast, the number of selected individuals who are absent decreases: in 2007, they represented 15.2% of the attempted contacts and in 2017 only 4.8%[11].

However, the most striking differences are observed at the level of the selection of households: 6.7% were not eligible in 2007 compared to 15.4% in 2017; also, the proportion of households where residents could not be found increased from 2.7% to 13.6%.

These developments together make the response rates in 2017, calculated relative to contacts established and to interviews requested, relatively comfortable.

Non-responses to specific survey questions

Despite the length of our questionnaire and the difficulty of the topic itself, interviewees fulfil the contract established in the interview relationship, if we consider that only 49 individuals did not answer all the questions; there is also the possibility that this number includes cases in which the incomplete information is due to the interviewer.

In general, respondents answer all questions. The rates of "non-response" or "don't know" are around 0.5% or, in some cases, 1% of the total. In fact, the distinction between the two categories does not always seem to be well grounded.

The exceptions are to be found, as in other studies, in the variables relating to income. In the case of own income, the answer "no answer" stands at 33.3% and "don't know" at 15.1%. These percentages are even higher when it comes to information on household income: 32.8% and 20.4% respectively. The other questions with the highest non-response rates are those concerning parents' level of education: between 9 and 11%.

On another level, questions on physical condition and health may also register non-response rates of between 3 and 6%.

As already mentioned, the degree of reliability that the interviewer attributes to information provided by interviewees is high. Even so, the sensitivity of the topics covered may explain that of the 77.4% of interviewees

[11] One can also discuss whether the number of retired people/pensioners may have some influence on this decrease in the number of missing selected individuals, as in 2007 the sample population was aged between 15 and 64 while in 2017 this had been extended to 74 years.

who are considered to provide good or very good information, only 28.8% fall into the "very good" bracket. It is undoubtedly exceedingly difficult to overcome concealment in an extensive interview relationship. We will therefore examine this issue in more detail in the following chapter, based on a source of intensive information.

Quality of interpretation and generalisation of results

Many of the questions related to the quality of the interpretation and the generalisability of the results are applied to surveys other than of the general population. Even so, we can take into account some specificities based on our own experience.

Processing errors

The multiple demands that public health priorities pose to surveys of the general population on the use of licit and illicit psychoactive substances, in addition to other non-substance addictive behaviours, require complex processing and database manipulation that are not common in smaller studies. On the other hand, part of the information has to be treated according to specifications and following parameters demanded by the needs of international comparison.

Furthermore, since this is a longitudinal study, the processing of information requires the analysis of different cohorts. This requires medium-term management of the results, with particular attention required in integrating them into narratives and models of understanding that correspond to different temporalities (political, social, cultural...). We shall illustrate some episodes associated with this type of concern in the last chapter of this section.

Also associated with this type of survey, some operations require careful attention at the processing stage, namely with the weightings and the processing conditions and possibilities that are allowed by the databases that result from them.

Inference errors

Where inference is concerned, as in any other type of survey, generalisations may be either too cautious or too ambitious. One of the advantages of probabilistic samples is that they allow us to calculate the margins of error of the results. Sometimes the readings are not comfortable, especially when they concern sensitive topics and problems that require rigorous information. On the part of researchers, it is a matter of not drawing unwarranted readings that the data do not justify. A recurrent tendency is to seek to validate readings on territories for which the results present considerable margins of error. This tendency is, however, difficult to counter, insofar as these are studies with a sample of unusual size but insufficient to provide information beyond the units for which it was formatted.

Still on the side of unwarranted readings, a form of causal inference, not constructed by the researchers, is by way of associating a certain result to the action of systems (namely in the field of public health) that the survey data is not in a position to validate... because these fields do not form a part of the observation protocols.

Probably the biggest inference problem that arises for surveys that, like ours, embrace a considerable set of behaviours is that they cannot justify reliable generalisations. Often the conditions of the studies, when these are focused on supporting the resolution of pressing problems, do not permit of processing in the medium term, or in the depth that would be desirable.

Conclusions

The above exposition confirms, it seems to us, that the construction of reality that the questionnaires allow—that is, the knowledge we can attain about the dimensions of the objects studied—results from the co-occurrence of multiple factors, and not only from the isolated efforts of research teams. This does not mean that the teams are relieved of any responsibility, but rather that their efforts should be framed within the contexts (political, scientific...) in which they operate. It also seems to us that the evaluation of the quality of the results obtained, particularly their validity or reliability, cannot be restricted to a definition of "errors" that—while they may occur and should be taken into account—do not permit of detailing all the operations that the researcher has to manage in order to arrive at the best possible knowledge of the object of study. Finally, this knowledge results from a dynamic process, in the sense that the variables that constrain it change over time and may produce unexpected effects, so that it cannot be found once and for all to be definitive.

We would like to think that the reference points that have guided us in this chapter, in conjunction with the further exposition below, may contribute to reflecting upon a matrix of the questions and dimensions that mark this process of clarification of hidden behaviours.

CHAPTER 2

DISSIMULATION IN DRUG USE RELATIONSHIP WITH PRIVACY AND CONSTRUCTION OF SPACES OF CONFIDENTIALITY

Presentation

Above we considered the capacity that questionnaires have to unveil, through the questions decided by the eye of the researcher, hidden dimensions of the characteristics of a population (while perhaps hiding others). We did not, however, look at the possible circumstance of this population not being available for this unveiling to take place. This w to hide, or to not allow the whole extension of a behaviour or all the nuances of a position to be seen, keeps away from the investigator's gaze precisely those objects that his questioning sought to show. This is to say that, in these cases, the dissimulation adds to the opacity inherent in observation.

Through survey methodology and checks on the reliability and validity of the questionnaires, the issue of measurement is traditionally resolved by adjusting the different procedures and instruments used so that they can capture as well as possible those objects that, although they may be dense or multi-dimensional, do not shy away from the observer's gaze. The hypothesis then formulated is that the observation instruments, if well calibrated, will eventually reduce the "measurement errors" that insinuate themselves between the observer and the observed and could thus be sources of biases between the observed and the observable. This concern with reducing measurement errors is at the basis of the effort with precautions and all the checks that accompany the collection operations that we detailed in the case of the INPG in the previous chapter. From this point of view of solving opacity problems, the issue of inaccurate information is resolved by appealing to a principle of random distribution of "lies" (in the declaration, for example, of a consumption behaviour) and considering that the probability of overstating is the same as that of understating, so that their effect is annulled. Short of any knowledge that we may have about the actual probability of this bias in the orientation of statements, the adoption of this principle corresponds more to a pragmatic position taken by the researcher, who thus eases the pressure from an area unknown to him, in order to accentuate the importance of the precautionary effort that he may in fact exert on the measurement conditions, in the form of the design and implementation of the questionnaire.

This precautionary effort is much more problematic when our aim is to acknowledge the effects on the results from survey situations in which the objects deliberately evade the investigator's gaze. We believe that this difficulty points, first of all, to the limits of the questionnaire as an instrument for extensive research, where it comes to finding out certain dimensions of the objects. However, these limits go beyond those that critics of extensive methods generally attribute to beliefs nurtured by a certain naïve positivism. Indeed, if the object hides from the observer and if their reasons for hiding are also sufficiently strong, then they will probably hide whatever the observation method used, including the most intensive approaches. It seems to us, however, that these intensive approaches, in accepting the loss of extension or representativeness, with what they gain in significance from an in-depth understanding of the objects can more easily attain knowledge of the strategies and reasons for concealment.

But what is dissimulation? And given that, by definition, individuals do not inform us that they are hiding something, how can we know if there is dissimulation when we gather a response from an informant? How do we decide that we are facing a situation of dissimulation when the criteria of "truth" may differ between actors and, even within the same actor, vary over time or through circumstances, namely the social relationship constructed to make the observation itself possible[12]? In addition, is it really the "truth" that is sought in a research process? Would it not be more reasonable to be content with the "truth" in which each subject bases the expression of their

[12] At this level, we believe that an interview relationship constructed to allow an intensive approach is in a better position to cope with concealment strategies than a more extensive approach (and within the latter, as we will see below, interview situations may vary greatly and decisively guide the results obtained).

identity in the present time (that is, at the moment of the interview), knowing as we do that individuals can reconstruct the meaning of their existences through time?

To try to answer these questions, we will develop the following reasoning:

- As a first step, we must identify both the main types of discourse that allow us to understand what dissimulation is and the modalities and forms in which secrecy and censorship may take shape in consumption relations. However, regardless of their modalities or forms, the meanings of dissimulation practices and strategies are influenced by multiple factors. We have isolated two of these factors that seem particularly relevant to us and which we shall present in the next two sections:
    - On the one hand, we shall consider the frameworks involved in setting the normative status of drug use and, more particularly, try to understand how they become normative benchmarks that allow individuals to rationalise their consumption behaviours and any dissimulation practices.
    - On the other hand, it seemed to us important to analyse the relationship that individuals establish with consumption and substances. In order to come closer to answering this question, we shall define different scenarios of consumption practices that present the places, in the literal and figurative senses, where and from which drug users dissimulate.
- Then, putting ourselves in the perspective of the individuals, we shall analyse the social relations of consumption, considering the main situations in which dissimulation may occur. These social relations of consumption, involving the various circumstances of their situations and individual idiosyncrasies, are anchored both in normative benchmarks and in consumption scenarios.
- In conclusion, we shall seek to explain the reasons why the meanings of dissimulation (and non-dissimulation), while generally transparent, may follow unpredictable strategies. We believe that the most compelling force of dissimulation strategies of is their plasticity.

Drug use and its relationship with "secrecy"

The concealment of consumption behaviour may be justified, beyond any protection of intimacy, by the legal interdiction that applies to the behaviour and, reinforcing this interdiction, by the social and moral disapproval that accompanies this. Given this normative and even moral burden that weighs on consumption, the first question we as researchers can ask is why someone who does not know me would respond to a survey interviewer, also unknown, who comes from who knows where and knocks on his door to ask if he "takes drugs". In fact, when this door-to-door approach is chosen[13], as in our case, it initially causes some perplexity, if not even a certain degree of anxiety, in the people who are contacted: "Why me, why such and such a person in my household?" We presume that an interview relationship that is built on such assumptions of normative and moral control and suspicion about the origin and objectives of the interlocutor is not conducive to the establishment of a relationship of trust likely to facilitate the full and unreserved communication of thc information requested. At least, we presume that this relationship is not as transparent as one that someone might have in the case where the object of the survey is the brand of soap used at home.

To identify, inventory and characterise drug use is, therefore, a somewhat paradoxical task, insofar as the aim is to clarify what society requires people to hide and what individuals have under normal conditions no interest in showing. But insofar as one accepts that this question may constitute an object of sociological study, it is a matter of mobilising the knowledge and tools of sociology to respond to the specific difficulties posed by such a study.

Having presented in the previous section the survey modalities that allow us to build the interview relationship, when it comes to the application of a questionnaire we are now interested in discussing the subjective reasons that individuals have to hide from others, and sometimes from themselves, the facts related to their consumption, or to reveal them only to those they consider can know them, so charting a circle of confidentiality.

In this section we intend to put these issues into perspective.

---

[13] We shall discuss in another chapter the choice of survey techniques and the effects they have on consumer statements.

Firstly, we must consider that the relationship with secrecy about consumption may vary over time. Undoubtedly, in a society where consumption is allowed, it would not be necessary to conceal it, or at least not for the same reasons as in a society that prohibits it. But where a given scenario of the social problem is concerned, different actors may have different discourses on consumption. We shall consider some that seem to us to be more relevant for our purposes. We shall then undertake a brief systematisation of the scientific literature on secrecy and then, finally, present the empirical material on which we shall base our analysis.

Universe of discourses on drug use

Types of discourse and evolution of a social problem

It is important to emphasise the changes that the problems of drug use have recorded during the last 20 years, to better frame the relationship between drug use and normative frameworks that, according to the hypothesis we formulated in the introduction, allows us to understand possible dissimulation on the part of drug users about behaviours that they know are stigmatising, culturally and socially.

In fact, the social problem of "drugs" and "addictions" has been reformulated following changes in the last two decades, to limit ourselves to the period that interests us here. These include: 1) the entry into the markets of new substances and changes in cultural patterns of use; 2) a new indexation of the importance of certain substances (greater importance given to tobacco or alcohol, for example) or non-substance-based dependence (gambling and the internet, etc.); 3) changes, also, in the growing attenuation of the gender effect on consumption, with women approaching men's levels[14]... These changes have been reflected in the orientations of successive SICAD Strategic Plans, which, although operating essentially under the legal framework of the decriminalisation law in force since the turn of the century, has been moulded to different institutional frameworks, with the framework currently in force defining

[14] The applications of the INPG (National survey on drug use among general population) between 2001 and 2016/17 make it possible to follow these changes (a synthesis of these results will be presented in *Vinte Anos de Consumo de Droga em Portugal*..., in preparation).

less integration between the levels of prevention and treatment than the previous one. At the same time, representations of public opinion on the social problems associated with consumption have also changed. For example, contrary to the situation at the beginning of the century, "drugs" do not appear in these representations as one of the country's most important problems[15].

A detailed analysis of these changes, taking into account, for example, how certain diagnoses are associated with certain actors, should show how the representations of the problems thus constructed are complex and open to a porous definition of the problems. They are complex, on the one hand, because these different representations tend to affirm irreconcilable points of view, motivated by different levels of intervention, supported by distinct centres or criteria of legitimacy and upheld by actors whose status may vary greatly. Although they tend to be formulated in the form of closed coherences, the circulation of these representations in the same space (despite, in certain cases, the inconsistency of their positions) opens up a field of uncertainty where the most diverse normative positions may be formulated. It is this dispersion of the possible that we sought to apprehend from the metaphor of "normative diffraction" (Balsa 2019). The interviews we shall analyse below show how drug users can find reasons for all their choices and legitimise them with socially anchored discourses.

Before going into their content orientations, it seems to us that discourses on consumption can be structured at the level of three distinct sensibilities: 1) on the one hand, we can consider the universe of professional discourses, when it comes to representations constructed by specialised agents in one of the different areas or levels of intervention associated with consumption; 2) at another level, we have the universe of securing discourses, which are produced by those—generally non-drug users—who construct representations that tend to work as modes of justification of individual conduct, balanced between the feeling of closeness and that of the distance that one wants to establish in relation to the universe of consumption and drug users; 3) finally, we can consider the

[15] A moral reading of the problem, supported by the great visibility that the most harmful situations of consumption had at the time, led public opinion to classify the "drug problem" as one of the country's most important, according to *O Estado da Nação — Data Crítica — Estudos de Opinião e Mercado* (2001, 12-14).

universe of legitimation discourses, which are constructed by drug users themselves and are intended to define the coherences, if not the rationality, that underlie their consumption practices.

It should be stressed that at the basis of these discourses are not necessarily individuals tied to the contingency of being "professionals", "drug users" or "non-drug users", but rather the statuses that individuals can take on, from which they rationalise situations and produce their representations.

Universe of professional discourses

The universe of professional discourses is constituted, as mentioned, by representations of specialised agents acting from any area or level of intervention related to consumption. By this we mean that the universe of professional discourses is constructed from the intersection of interventions legitimated by a certain area of knowledge and intervention and by certain spaces of activity or institutional places. We were able to analyse discourses of this type in the case of professionals—representatives of employers' associations, trade unions, public entities and large companies—involved with the problems of consumption associated with the work environment. In this case, what is at stake is the attribution of responsibilities regarding the consequences that consumption may have at various levels: profitability and business costs, the working conditions imposed, workers' health and safety, risks to third parties, for example, through the services provided by companies. Our work on consumption in the workplace allowed us to list the numerous dimensions from which these types of representations can be constructed (Balsa, Urbano and Vital 2021).

Universes of securing discourses

Portugal's national survey on drug use among general population includes several batteries of questions that seek to obtain knowledge about the universes of discourses of individuals based, essentially, on an estimate of risks associated with different substances. These batteries are aimed at the whole population—drug users and non-drug users—thus avoiding a situation where the survey is conducted exclusively around the construction of an individual consumer and drug addict. The reason for this orientation lies in the fact that since this is a "national survey" and targets the "general population" it is necessary to open up the dimensions of the representations in order to be able to consider individuals whatever their orientation towards consumption. Besides this reason, which is linked to the very object of the survey, we could invoke another one of a more pragmatic nature that has to do with the fact that the aim is to make the most, in terms of the information collected, of a survey a large number of individuals (around 12,000 per application) of whom only relatively small proportions (in the case of some substances, even very small proportions) declare their use of illicit substances. This means that, for the vast majority of the population, we collect above all information on the representations of risks on the part of individuals who do not consume.

It is in this sense that the INPG allows us to access the universe of securing discourses—that is to say, a delimitation of the risks that individuals are unwilling to take—formulated by those who do not consume. The results of this risk mapping are discussed in the reports of the successive applications of the Study and will be the object of a synthesis in the book on 20 years of drug use in Portugal (in preparation).

Universes of discourses of legitimation

In the same way that the National Survey allows us to analyse the representations of non-drug users, it also allows us to analyse the positions of those who declare some consumption. We note, moreover, that consumption behaviours may coincide with restrictive representations of the risks that may be associated with them. However, as we said, the extensive and generalising approach is not the most appropriate to apprehend the meanings of consumption, beyond their most external dimensions. Therefore, in the case of drug users, an approach is justified which enables us to reconstruct discourses from the individuals' own reasons and not, as is the case of surveys using questionnaires, from dimensions *a priori* aimed at filling out epidemiological tables.

The focus on the universe of discourses of legitimation thus motivated a specific approach, in the form of in-depth interviews that, while conducted according to a "script" that translates our research concerns, always left open a space that individuals could shape according to their specific experiences and their own system of priorities. It is these discourses of legitimation that we will look at in this chapter.

Figures of secrecy and situations of censorship

Secrecy represents the informant's ability or prerogative not to talk, not to talk enough, or to talk too much, in most cases in order to keep quiet about what they see as essential. André Petitat (2014) has highlighted the dimensions that shape this prerogative and defined the modalities under which it presents itself. The effects of communication understood through the reading grid that is ESCO (space of secrecy and ordinary knowledge) would thus represent a particular modality—which implies the intentionality of the subject—of the usual resistance offered by the objects of sociology to observation. André Petitat (Petitat, n.d.) considers that this intentionality constructs the social relation from three places: 1) visibility (showing or hiding oneself); 2) metamorphosis (deforming one's experience or transmitting it in authentic form); and 3) normativity (respecting or transgressing the rules of communication).

According to the decisions taken from each of these places, three figures of concealment take shape that play out on the axis of trust/distrust that regulates communication (Petitat 1996, 1; n.d, 7 and 12):

- the lie (hidden/transformed/illegitimate);
- the unsaid (hidden/not transformed/illegitimate);
- intimacy and discretion (hidden/not transformed/legitimate).

The "lie" occurs when information is illegitimately transformed (from the perspective of conventional communication codes); the "not said" when, in illegitimate fashion, it is hidden by omission; and "intimacy or discretion" when the omission may be considered to be legitimate, as far as events considered to be in the domain of people's intimacy are concerned.

These figures overlap and inform other figures of concealment that may not require the mobilisation of the individuals' intentionality, and which occur beyond a situation of formal communication. Among these the author considers the unknown, the ambiguous, the misunderstood, the mystery, the secret from oneself, the illusion, the convenience, the allusion, the misunderstanding, the ideology and the rationalisation.

Where the dissimulation of hidden behaviours is concerned, we are mainly interested in understanding secrecy in a situation in which the concealment is aimed at an entity or person who is considered to be able to reprimand or punish the consumption behaviours on the basis of any of the orders for judgement that may be mobilised. In other words, the practice of secrecy always exists in relation to a censorship that the subject acknowledges but whose normative injunction they are not willing to follow, at least not immediately.

Censorship thus manifests itself when an entity addresses the subject from the outside, preventing them from saying or doing everything that they would be disposed to say or do. In this sense, we may consider different modalities of censorship, from "commission", which is responsible for controlling discourses, to the different orders of censorship that are exercised, with different degrees of formality and coercive power, in the name of the principles on the basis of which they are established. In the case of consumption, these orders are derived from a health, legal or moral judgement. The law constrains consumption by limiting its acceptability from the point of view of health and individual responsibility. The different instances of censorship may in some cases intervene only implicitly based on the internalisation, by the agents, of their respective normative frameworks. In P. Bourdieu's expression, perfect censorship, which is in fact invisible, is exercised when the agent has nothing more to say than what he has been previously authorised to say (Bourdieu 1977).

Censorship and secrecy, or rather, censoring entities and the ESCO (space of secrecy and ordinary knowledge), thus always constitute two moments associated with the process of concealment. Any expression, states P. Bourdieu (ibid. 1977, 385), always results from an expressive interest and a censorship constituted by the structure of the field that allows this expression. The euphemisation effort, which aims to adapt what is said to what can be said, may go as far as silence, the limiting case of a censored discourse.

In the case of declarations of consumption in a formal interview situation, which we are interested in analysing here, in addition to the countless situations through which strategies of secrecy are implemented, the explicit reference to an instance of censorship occurs when someone being interviewed, who is therefore ready to reveal their consumption to the interviewer, says that they are unavailable to conduct the interview at home, to avoid family members overhearing who would not approve of them[16].

We can thus see that individuals may restrict their circles of confidentiality according to the orientation of the normative orders with which they are confronted. It seems equally plausible to us, to follow P. Bourdieu's reasoning, that these normative orders are indexed to fields within which their modes of imposition and legitimacy are defined. We acknowledge, however, that each field may be affected by several normative orders. Thus, for example, friends may be confidants, but on condition that they share the same consumption "culture"; indeed, friends with whom knowledge of a particular consumption is shared may be excluded from knowledge of the consumption of other substances. On another level, the natural visibility of a consumption when performed in its usual context can be broken by the intrusion of an unexpected gaze that sees what "it should not have seen".

These orientations lead us to believe that there is no unambiguous relationship between the strategies and reasons for confidentiality, on the one hand, and the circumstances of space, time and social relations in which they are applied, on the other.

We seek to analyse these reasons and strategies of secrecy below, but first we present the empirical approach on which we rely.

Presentation of empirical approach and of discourses analysed

According to A. Petitat (Petitat 1996, 1; n.d, 7 and 12) the ideal of scientific knowledge presupposes: 1) the object's total transparency; 2) the methods' total adequacy; and 3) absolute respect of the conventions that regulate the interrelationships or, at least, total transparency of the transgression strategies that may be adopted by the subjects in cases where the observation of the facts is not direct. The research product always results from a compromise between these three types of obstacles. This is why the scientific ideal, which we portray here according to Jean Ladrière's

[16] This possibility can, in fact, be countered by interview techniques in two ways: 1) on the one hand, the use of CAPI (computer-assisted personal interviewing), which ensures that people who do not belong to the technical team cannot access the questionnaire content; 2) on the other, the use of cards, so that that the names of the substances are never verbalised.

definition (Piaser and Ladrière 1976), is not achieved in a definitive way, but rather is outlined in a distant horizon, through an effort of constant adaptation, between an *a priori* normativity, because the scientific discourse has to obey rules that distinguish it from others, and a constantly renewed facticity, resulting from the confrontation of the rules with the always singular data of each research. From the perspective of observation, what is at stake here, in addition to seeking to bring the observed as close as possible to the observable, whose status is virtual, is arriving at knowledge of the scenarios that make the data collected intelligible from the perspective of the observed subject and the communication strategies he may adopt, taking into account the dynamics of the normative contexts that constrain the observation.

The universe of the experiences studied

Our empirical approach was undertaken exclusively with users of illicit psychoactive substances. The selection of interviewees was made following a quota system, requiring proportionality between men and women and the types of substances consumed. Thus, 37 people were interviewed with the following profile[17]:

- Gender: 15 females and 22 males;
- Age: minimum 18, maximum 44, with an average age of 28;
- Dominant substances at time of interview or last used (almost all interviewees have used several substances in their lives, often simultaneously):
    - heroin: 8
    - cocaine: 8
    - ecstasy: 5
    - hallucinogens: 6
    - cannabis: 10

---

[17] We are grateful for the valuable contributions of Miguel Chaves and the researchers who were then part of the team at CEOS, Investigações Sociológicas, NOVA FCSH. We would also like to thank the teams who conducted the interviews and transcribed them. Finally, we thank the people who agreed to reconstruct their experiences of consumption. They opened up to us the complexity of our object of study and allowed us to find out about their "secrets". Their information was fundamental for us to understand the circumstances in which they would not answer a questionnaire.

Interviews were carried out following a mixed administration technique that provided for the application of a script structured around the research themes, but which at the same time allowed scope for discovery when the interviewee's experience did not fit into the lines of the script. Apart from a small form for gathering some individual details (such as gender and age, household composition, means of subsistence, sociability networks, and school and professional experiences), the interviews focussed on three central topics:

- consumption practices;
- relationship with substances; and
- relationships of confidentiality.

The corpus that resulted from transcription of the interviews consists of 852 pages. Each interview is identified by a serial number and, when deemed necessary, we indicate some of the characteristics of the person interviewed.

Construction and analysis of the corpus

The analysis was carried out by the joint use of two techniques: 1) a classification by category, aimed at inventorying the themes and constructing the space of the dimensions that corresponded to the set of experiences reported; and 2) the construction of significant isotopies of the main meanings of the individual positions and of the orientations of the cultural models they denote in relation to the topics targeted by the study.

To reduce the length of the text, we have limited our references to interviews to the excerpts that seem to us to best represent the meaning of the categories analysed. Interviews are identified by the arbitrary serial number that they have in the corpus, and, within each interview, excerpts are identified by the response number. In the transcripts, we kept marks that might be relevant for the understanding of the positions analysed, but corrected errors and eliminated redundancies typical of oral expression.

Normative orders and references of consumption

Among the discourses mentioned above, we are interested here in deepening those that aim at legitimation, which are, in fact, the only ones we can process based on the materials we analyse. To this end, we shall first of all identify the main normative orders that apply to consumption. Then, based on our material, we shall be in a position to understand how individuals appropriate these orders to build normative references that will serve them to decide, manage and evaluate their consumption.

Normative orders

Unlike most of the other objects available in the market whose consumption is essentially regulated by subjective criteria (need, taste...), social status or economic power, the use of psychoactive substances, especially those defined as illicit, is also indexed to norms that are usually well codified by institutions that define the possibilities of consumption or that, in some way, regulate them, through devices or instruments of a more or less coercive character, according to the nature of the institutions or the targeted substances. This means that in order to approximate knowledge of existing normative frameworks (which are not always perfectly codified as is the case with the legal framework) we must consider the action of the agents who are in some way charged with putting them forward or imposing sanctions for their non-observance (cf. Becker 1985).

The three main instances of normative production that we feel should be considered are: the legal, the medical and the moral. The orientations of these normative frameworks have varied over time, with a shift having been observed on the part of some of the criteria for evaluating the status of consumption or its consequences — a process that has been well studied by analysts (cf. in particular, Balsa 2020). At the legal level, we know that the decriminalisation of certain consumption has led to policies of prevention and monitoring (medical, psychological, social...) tailored to technical diagnoses of situations, thus expanding the range of responses to the problem, which were previously essentially repressive. This change coincided with a new evaluation, in the field of health, of the physical and psychological effects of drug use, allowing dependence to be classified as a disease and treated as such, and intervention strategies to be implemented that focus on prevention and on the principle of the reduction of harms associated with drug use. To what extent do these changes alter the moral discourse based on the opposition between the "good" of abstinence and the "evil" represented by consumption? The information we are handling here does not allow us to answer these questions directly. These different normative orders are, however, mobilised by our interviewees, who use them to construct the discourses through which they legitimise their positions relative to consumption. For example, we do not know to what extent the shift from the criminal paradigm to a health paradigm was internalised by the different orders under consideration, but we can find out how the discourse attributed to these orders is perceived by individuals and how they appropriate these perceptions to construct their own rationalities towards the established discourse. For example: "The conclusion was reached that drug addiction was a disease... there you are, it's not bad any more, although I think there are many people who don't see it that way, not at all...". (E11/R117). Or here: "The police still think a bit like they used to: if a person is a drug addict, he's a criminal... and doctors, of course, know that it's a disease, don't they?" (E13/R202).

It is on the basis of how the orientations in place are represented and appropriated that we can construct the discourses of legitimation, from the level of individuals, that concern us here.

We may attempt a first approximation at these normative orders by singling out two dimensions that seem to us may constitute them[18]: 1) on the one hand, the way the law is internalised by individuals, in which we can distinguish two limiting cases: the norm is taken on in its generic aspects and consequences or, on the contrary, is subject to some reservation or interpretation; 2) on the other, the very consumption behaviours that are the object of the norm and which individuals may or may not feel the need to dissimulate. The subdivision we can make of these dimensions allows us to separate out four typological orientations[19]:

---

[18] As always, typological approaches allow classifications that only help us to better understand certain aspects of the realities studied but can neither limit nor simplify the complexity of the positions that make up that reality.

[19] This substruction draws on the one that Merton constructed to analyse the types of adaptation by individuals to society (Merton, Robert k. 1965. "Structure sociale, anomie et déviance." In *Déviance et criminalité*, pp. 132-165. Textes réunis par Denis Szabo. Paris: Librairie Armand Colin, 1970, 378 pp. Collection "U/U2"

Typology of normative referentials		**Relation with the prohibition norm**	
		Incorporated	Not incorporated
Disclosure of consumption behaviours	Non-dissimulation	Conformity	Counter-normative
	Dissimulation	Dissonance	Diffraction

Discourses of legitimation can thus be organised around these different modal positions—which we shall call normative referentials—which articulate in a specific way the normative orders that frame consumption. We shall detail the following:

- normative conformity referential;
- normative dissonance referential;
- normative diffraction referential;
- referential counter-normative;
- anomie referential.

We are not interested here in analysing these referentials as such, focusing on their possible internal coherence; rather, we are interested in when they are perceived through the social relations in which individuals participate, which we shall designate, based on the materials we analyse, as social relations of consumption. This relational dimension is maintained even when we refer to the situation of people living alone, who are always confronted not only with their own evaluations but also with the evaluation of their behaviours by some instance of social censorship.

(http://classiques.uqac.ca/contemporains/Merton_RobertK/Structure_soc_anomie_deviance/Structure_soc_anomie_deviance_texte.html).

Normative referentials

Normative conformity referential

It seems to us reasonable to think that, regardless of the more or less nuanced way it is done, or the deferral strategies through which it is done, the three normative orders that we have been considering—the legal, the health and the moral—point to abstinence from all consumption as the right way to achieve the values or resources that they proclaim: order, health and goodness. The question that we may then ask ourselves is to what extent these orders are accepted, internalised and have consequences on the positions that individuals adopt. If we consider the discourses we analyse from the perspective of the values that dominate the three orders mentioned—and which are guided by the principle of abstinence—we may define a referential of normative conformity when the representations of individuals are in line with the orientations that these orders impose; this means that individuals adopt them, if not to regulate their behaviours, at least to evaluate them.

At first sight, this position presents us with a paradox: insofar as the reference population considered here is made up of drug users, those normative orders have indeed been violated. We can then consider the issue from two different angles.

From the users' perspective, a normative compliance referential presents itself, in the first place, as an external injunction, either through the discourses of institutions, particularly of any of its instances (police, medical or moral), or through the position of a significant other (family members, for example). In our material, this referential is better apprehended in the negative, that is, when it is referred to in the discourses of drug users as an external constraint that they cannot ignore and against which they generally position themselves.

However, the normative conformity referential may also be acknowledged by the drug users themselves; in these cases, it essentially leads to situations of cognitive dissonance that express, in the drug users themselves, a conflict between being a consumer and the duty not to be: *"I say [people] shouldn't use drugs and I do, but that's up to each person... I think the trip itself is a drug that — I don't say all people should try, but most people should, because it brings something different to life, I don't know, man... Sometimes it's good, sometimes it's bad... But I think a normal person should try it. I mean just try it, I don't mean to keep taking it."* (E36/R99).

We can observe situations of cognitive dissonance in two very different scenarios: 1) when consumption starts, when it can still be considered an accident without meaning in a path that many think will be without drugs — a feeling that is, in fact, confirmed in approximately two thirds of the individuals who declare that they have experimented with drugs; and 2) in a phase of consumption in which nothing can be hidden any longer.

The referential of conformity, while it cannot be ignored at the moment of first consumption, can however intervene in different ways, from situations in which the individual was unaware of committing an illicit act to multiple situations in which other reasons (the desire to experiment or group solidarity...) prevailed over normative considerations (see below). There are, nevertheless, cases in which consumption occurred despite being frowned upon: *"At the time I was even a little against the use of drugs, of hashish. I had the idea that it was dangerous, and I didn't feel like trying it"* (E12/R42); *"I was against it, always against it, not hashish, I am against that... I don't smoke any of that"* (E35/R57); *"One of the reasons why I had broken up with him was because he used drugs — I realised it was hashish. And to make me understand that it was harmless, he gave me some to try."* (E11/R9).

Another very different situation of cognitive dissonance is observed at the end of a consumption path gone wrong, when its consequences lead drug users to desire the norm of abstinence against the "world of drugs" that they consider to be a world without values: *"This world is a bit like that, there are no friends, there are no values, there is nothing, anything goes... I'm fed up, I'm fed up, fed up with drugs right now... If they told me 'You have the opportunity to go to your father's house for a week, to be with your daughters'... I wouldn't think twice."* (E11/R45).

We can thus see that the situations in which consumption coincides with an alignment to a normative conformity referential are observed before the installation of consumption routines, or else when these routines are experienced as a burden to be borne and of which individuals aim to rid themselves. In both cases, the concealment of consumption is not necessary. Experimental use can be admitted without serious consequences; sometimes, this use is known to those around them and tolerated; often, what is hidden is not this experimental use but the routine use of less accepted substances that follows. Sometimes, even, confessing to experimental use serves as a smokescreen to hide the other kind. Meanwhile, people with substances use disorders and those in the rejection phase, generally no longer have anything to hide.

However, in most situations of established use, in which individuals declare some capacity to manage it (cf. below, consumption situations), they construct rationales that allow them to justify and maintain their consumption, against the guidelines of the dominant normative referential. These rationalisations will follow modulations of positioning that can be better understood by employing the other referentials we have listed.

Normative dissonance referential

Consumption behaviours in contexts that censor consumption lead at the very least to biased social relations, when the individual has to hide consumption from others, so trying to avoid or mitigate some consequence—material, social, but especially moral—that the revelation of his behaviour could have. This bias is the basis of a second referential that we will call cognitive dissonance. In the normative dissonance referential, there is a divergence of positions in relation to the norm of abstinence, but only to the extent of compliance or non-compliance with abstinence, that is, of behaviour: the norm itself is not directly brought into question. In fact, this norm intervenes in the relationship in transfigured form, through two modes of filtering. On the one hand, it intervenes in the discourse in the way in which it is attributed to an authority that supposedly upholds it. Here, the contestation of the norm is indirect and always mediated by the contestation of that authority, and it is therefore not necessary to construct a discourse of opposition to the norm itself: *"In all public institutions there's a kind of discourse... It is a memorised discourse... So, there's no point in talking to them."* (E6/R126) At another level, the abstinence norm is put into perspective: it is not the abstract norm itself that is questioned, and which can even, at this level, be considered adequate, but a formulation considered to be adulterated (for example, "hypocritical" (E12/R94)) that is attributed to the discourse or practices of some source of authority: *"What you hear in the media are the negative aspects, always, which is to influence people not to consume... But it's not 100% true! I think it's even good because people shouldn't consume... But I know that beyond that there's always something else that's good."* (E36/R98) In the same way, the idea of conformity may be brought into question that is conveyed by the position of parents, for example.

The cognitive dissonance referential can be observed in all situations of consumption that require its reporting, i.e., that imply asymmetric social relations (work environment, family environment, institutional environments) attributing different statuses and levels of subordination to the respective partners, associated with different levels of constraint: from a simple relationship of respect [*"My grandmother is already old, if she knew I think she would be very sad... I think that there are some cases where it's maybe better not to say anything about it!"* (E12/R100)] to even physical constraint [*"Once, my father put a pistol to my head and told me that if I ever got deep into drugs, he would shoot me. And he said that if he had to have a son who was a junkie he'd rather have a son who was dead first, at least he would only suffer grief once."* (E15/R230)]. In the absence of this asymmetric relationship, the issue of dissonance does not arise, either because the consumer does not have to report his behaviour to anyone, or because he can himself impose his reasoning as a consumer on someone; naturally, the latter case would lead to relationships of conflict, precisely the outcome that drug users tend to avoid or postpone. One of the ways of doing this is to face up to the dissonance, by concealing the existence of the behaviours before the significant others in the relationship. From the consumer's point of view, this type of relationship thus opens up a strategy space, involving, on the one hand, the adoption of dissimulation modalities according to the game of reciprocal expectations and, on the other, the production or mobilisation of resources appropriate to the need to hide.

Also in this referential, there is the relationship with consumption that is better understood based on the figure of foreclusion, i.e. when, before seeking to conceal consumption from others, the consumer tends to hide it from himself. This self-dissimulation seems to function as a first bulwark of the strategy of dissimulation to others (and is probably a way of mitigating the possible effects of cognitive dissonance).

Normative diffraction referential

A third normative referential may also be considered when drug users, unable to escape the imposition of the prohibitionist norm, even if they intend to ignore it, seek to shape it in line with their consumption experiences and according to the consumption legitimation effects that they seek to obtain. We shall speak, in these cases, of a *normative diffusion referential*[20]*:* there is no clear delimitation of the contours of the norm when it is received by its addressees.

While in the dissonance referential the normative divergences are materialised in the people or institutions that supposedly embody the norm, in this referential it is the norm itself that is targeted in the discourse, through its reinterpretation and translation, in order to make acceptable certain consumptions (but not others...) or their circumstances or modalities. Insofar as this rationalisation is not shared with significant others (through cultures or subcultures of consumption, for example), the dissimulation of consumption allows the relations deemed necessary or significant for drug users to be maintained (while perhaps abandoning some others).

The diffraction of the norm occurs when it is reinterpreted, for example by relativising the importance or relevance of the normative framework that imposes and regulates it, calling into question the relevance of its object (illicit substances are no more dangerous than licit ones...) or its scope (everyone takes drugs).

In a relationship context dominated by a normative conformity referential, it becomes very difficult to reconcile the defence of an abstinence principle and the existence of a consumption practice. This is undoubtedly due to the firm conviction rooted in the referential of conformity of the goodness and natural universality recognised in the principle of abstinence. This conviction makes it very difficult for those who profess it to accept a consumption behaviour.

However, if we consider the socio-institutional level itself, where the referentials of abstinence are produced, we see that it is possible to relativise this principle of abstinence to justify, for example, a policy of reduction of harms caused by consumption. This means that in these cases the norm is still abstinence but, considering a certain set of circumstances (such as a

[20] We have developed this figure of "normative diffraction" in another paper (cf. Balsa 2020).

relative banalisation of the use of certain substances in certain categories of the population and the evident failure, in these cases, of prohibitionist policies), the option is taken to relativise the coercive and general character of the norm, framing it in an alternative reading appropriate to the aims in view: to reduce harms caused by consumption. Insofar as the ideal of abstinence continues to impose itself, or so long as it remains important in some institutional environments with responsibilities for regulating the issue of consumption, harm reduction policies will themselves be diffractive in relation to the prohibitionist norm.

In terms of individual rationalisations, this retranslation of the abstinence principle always leads to the legitimisation of a certain level or type of consumption. The general principle of this position is precisely to construct an alternative narrative that makes consumption acceptable from the consumer's perspective. This is achieved, not by contesting the foundations of the norm (as the counter-normative referential will do), but by perverting, one by one, its assumptions.

A diffractive form of reading consists in challenging the scientific knowledge that can support the prohibition principle, opposing it to the knowledge that comes from the experience of consumption: *"The effects that drugs have on me"* (E31/R111). The scientific method is further questioned because it would not allow the achievement of convergent results (*"There are doctors who use a method to study drugs that others do not use and come to different conclusions, and then there are those contradictions"*, ibid.) or because its assumptions are contested (*"The quality of the sample... maybe the quality of the drugs they are testing and the experimental conditions..."*, ibid.). This causes doctors to come to opposite conclusions: *"The other day I read a Dutch doctor saying that for him cocaine was not considered a drug and that anyone could do cocaine three times a week (laughs)"* (Ibidem). Furthermore, the prohibitionist discourse is not coherent with the practice of doctors who themselves prescribe 'drugs': *"They are the main agents in promoting drug use... For example, psychiatrists, in this case, deal mostly with drugs, don't they? With the administration of legal drugs, much stronger than hashish, for example"* (E30/R93).

At another level, the legitimacy of the institutions that promote the interdiction of consumption is also questioned. Thus, *"people give full credit to doctors"*, but a 'shaman' *"could inform more about any psychedelic drug, you know?"* (E31/R111). This legitimacy may also not be recognised to the instances of control [*"There have been cops... who were arrested for drug trafficking and after two or three weeks they were out..."* (E15/R239)] or the "government" itself: *"But the government also, if you don't mind my saying, they also get involved there, because they really have to, and there are certain kinds of situations that everyone who knows about thinks twice"* (Ibidem). The bodies promoting the moral order are also targeted: *"Religious figures are in the same game of hypocrisy as the state and so it's not worth it"* (E6/R128).

The principle of the abstinence norm can also be questioned from the relevance of its purposes: 1) the defence of the common interest is contested because consumption would be the rule and not the exception that one wants to combat: *"Everybody consumes!"* (E20/R54); *"The first time and the second time I experimented it was with a doctor... You see, doctors also give it out... Even in the government, man!"* (E6/R117); 2) the scope of the very law that decriminalises drug use is also targeted, with the view that use without trafficking is legal [*"I think the illegal thing isn't using, the illegal thing is trafficking"* (E20/R398)]; 3) the selection of prohibited substances is considered arbitrary [*"Smoking hashish occasionally, or even coke, or even heroin and, well, everything, I mean those are substances like other medicinal substances and less dangerous even"* (E12/R94); *"It is proven that smoking a joint does less harm than smoking a cigarette, you know? Drinking a coffee is worse than smoking a joint. So, this is scientific data, but socially and culturally people do not assimilate this"* (E6/R61)].

Finally, the alignment of the norm with some of the social values it aims to promote can also be questioned. Thus, on the one hand, the relevance attributed to the prohibitionist norm in the integration of individuals and the defence of the integrity of their identities is denied [*"Using does not change anything"* (E33/R79)]: 1) when one does not consume in order to do something [*"That's the problem, that is I think that a guy who is aiming for something through drugs is the guy who can most easily end up addicted"* (E31/R68)]; and, 2) one does not stop doing something because there are no substances [*"If I want to go to a party I go anyway, I don't need to consume to go there"* (E10/R113)]. On the other hand, questioning any rationale associated with the prohibition of use, namely, the definition of dependence as a health problem: *"Those guys who create these stigmas... They really don't know what it is or what it isn't!"* (E33/R134); the issue of consumption can only be considered from the perspective *"always, of personal freedom"* (E33/R135). Consumption is regulated only by individual responsibility, since *"drugs depend on people's heads!"* (E33/R53).

Counter-normative referential

We can also consider a fourth referential, when we are faced with a situation in which the injunction of abstinence and the normative frameworks that defend it are directly challenged, creating the possibility of a counter-normative referential that, in its full expression, would signify a position that defends the justness or legitimacy of consumption.

Certainly, the different types of retranslation with which the norm is confronted in the previous referentials already signify, in fact, ways of circumventing the principle of abstention, some playing on the codes and others on the authorities that impose them. In the counter-normative referential, norms and values are equally brought into question in the name of an alternative rationality.

The best way of understanding this referential is to understand its relationship with the values that define it. Rather than going against the prohibitionist discourse, it is a matter here of associating it with a political logic that would give it meaning: *"Society is a society of cognitive censorship... The state prohibits certain types of states of consciousness, but nevertheless allows others..."* (E31/R110). This selective permissiveness is not random, but based on a choice: *"The state is doing its job... I understand the state's position (despite all the hypocrisy) ... in prohibiting"* (ibid.). This legitimacy would be based less on morality (*"LSD was a drug that the CIA was testing on young people"* [E31/110]) and would be supported more by an economic logic: *"If people all took LSD, nobody would bother to work"* (E31/110). It is, therefore, an economic logic that would be the basis of prohibition: *"New York and all the stock markets work on that basis"*; *"Maybe the state might as well sell caffeine, and meat, and sugar, and all those stimulants... And cocaine itself"* (ibid).

Placed thus in this perspective, the legitimacy of the norm becomes relative, and it is possible to accept or refuse it. Acceptance is attributed to people's ignorance: *"The state knows what substances do to people but, and in the case of Portugal, they know that people are ignorant, people are not prepared to receive certain types of information"* (Ibidem). However, knowledge can lead to refusing that legitimacy: *"That makes it possible for you not to accept what the state says and to recognise a parallel state"* (Ibidem): *"It's like this: I don't live by the rules of this government, or any government, at all. I live by my own rules, my government is me!"* (E20/R259).

At the level of behaviours, the most abrupt expression of this opposition would take the form of defending the absence of restrictions on the use of any substance, regardless of the injunctions not to consume. This limiting case can be observed: *"They may not legalise it, it doesn't matter to me! It may be prohibited, or lead to prison, but I couldn't give a s***. If I walk past a police station and feel like smoking a joint, I'll smoke it outside the police station! I know I'm going to get done, I know they're going to beat me..."*. (E20/R259). However, the counter-normative position tends to reject the norm of abstinence for certain substances, namely for the recreational use of cannabis in its different varieties. This orientation is sometimes adopted based on their own experience, or the experience of friends or family, of using other substances: *"I give a lot of importance to people who were the heroin generation... who lived with hallucinogenic drugs, in a huge boom, which was all out of control and who also later were lost because of a lack of information"* (E31/R113).

Anomie referential

We have also collected material that allows us to construct a position beyond those that fit our substruction (see table above). In this new position, normative frameworks based on the principle of abstinence are called into question, but without their being countered with diffractive or, much less, counter-normative readings. In these positions, the dominant normative frameworks simply cease to exist. We are confronted here, less with the situation of "anarchy" claimed in the reading proposed by one of our interviewees (E3/R217) than with an anomie referential: normative frames of reference can simply no longer be mobilised to regulate individual behaviours[21].

The account of two consumption situations allows us to better understand this position. In the first case, our interviewee brought into question the relevance of what he was asked, arguing that it had nothing to do with his world as a consumer: *"But I don't know what you want... What do I say? I don't know what you want, man... People take drugs and they don't know why!"* (E5/R192). Addiction (in this case rejected) leads to consumption, despite all the circumstances that could result in not using: *"Do you think one likes to do that? Do you think it was nice? It wasn't nice. Hey, man, listen, I don't understand what you ... it's a matter of... it's really s***, [interviewer's name] ... That's why I'm saying that whoever did this [the questions] has never consumed!"* (E5/R192-3).

In fact, although the script was conducted following the principle of empathic listening, empathy is a process that is built throughout the interview and, when it is achieved, the results only truly appear at the moment of analysis. But, after the analysis, the researcher is not only confronted with the "world of a consumer", but also with the worlds of all the drug users interviewed, from which he hopes, as we do here, to build totalisations that fit as closely as possible the universe of the experiences collected... In this sense, in a certain way, our interviewee is right in reading the world of drugs on the basis of the idea of "anarchy", if this can be interpreted as a universe fractured by multiple reasons and rationalities and where each one of them is only valid for the circumstances that surround them. But through all these cases, individuals try to construct their reasons... In the cases that interest us here, the search for reasons is rejected, with the inevitability imposed by the need to consume being invoked in its place. Sometimes, individuals seek to distance themselves from their relationship with consumption [*"People take drugs and they don't know why!"* (E5/192)]; in other cases, they view themselves as subjects of that relationship (blaming an "addiction" or a "habit").

On the normative level, normative frameworks may even be rejected: *"I don't care about anything. I don't vote, I don't care about politics, I detest*

---

[21] We update here a classification of normative positions that we developed in another work and in another domain of action where positions took forms around three modal positions: normative, alternative and counter-normative (Balsa 2002).

*politics! I've heard so much about this country, such a load of crap, you know? On every subject, not only drugs... I'm talking about every aspect... that I don't even care! They're clowns that are there talking ... they only talk s***."* (E20/R253) However, this rejection of order is not countered with any alternative: it only represents the claim of a specific meaning for a singular space of consumption. That means that these positions do not fit into a counter-normative referential. Beyond a counter-normative position, the absence of order means, in these cases, anomie.

This figure of anomie thus appears in conjunction with situations of dependence (those that were observed were outside any kind of institutional support) and in some cases these appear associated with experiences of trafficking or other illegal activities linked to obtaining the means to acquire substances. As will be better documented below, these experiences are related to a clear absence of moral values, when practices among the users themselves are mentioned. In these latter cases the accounts we collected, although they may nurse hopes of a different world, are presented to us as a manifestation of complaint: in the most extreme situations of dependence, often the relationship with normativity does not go beyond the horizon of the very life circumstances in which the consumption occurs.

Conclusions

Some clarifications are necessary in order to situate the status of the positioning orientations that we have just presented.

Firstly, none of these referentials exhausts the positioning possibilities of individuals, although according to the consumption scenarios (cf. below) and the nature of the social relations in which they are involved, some are more likely than others. This also means that the same narrative of legitimisation may mobilise different referentials.

Secondly, insofar as these positions are analysed here based on individual discourses of legitimisation (cf. above) focused on a particular consumption scenario, they are always signified based on a partial and fragmentary mobilisation of normative orders of reference: a discourse that articulates legal, health and moral order requires on the part of the person interviewed an analytical competence that is difficult to organise in the course of an interview. Despite this, and also because of this, this type of mobilisation makes it possible to identify the referentials that individuals utilise to assess the conformity or nonconformity of their consumption. However, while these referentials offer the criteria for this assessment at the individual level, they do not immediately constitute any instance of reporting. This means that normative positions can only be constructed and signified within a social relationship that will take on a certain role according to the positions that its different actors adopt in relation to normative orders. Thus, the decision to hide or not to hide arises when consumer behaviour is confronted with the provisions of legal codes, health guidelines or society's expectations, based on certain moral values. But before any possible outcome, this confrontation imposes the decision to hide or not to hide as the result of a social relationship, and it is only based on the density, but also on the unpredictability that this social relation brings, that the positions of individuals can be perceived. The next step is therefore to determine at what levels or to what entities the individuals are, by some moral imperative or social constraint, made accountable, and what the modalities of this accountability mean for their positions. At a first level, the statements collected translate the positions that individuals wished to assert in the interview relationship, and only at a second level do they reveal the way in which relationships may be resolved with other significant persons for individuals and the circumstances that will always constrain them.

Finally, considering the referential in the perspective of social relationships and possible strategies of dissimulation, it is clear that one way of avoiding biases in relationships that may be associated with any of the situations analysed is to suspend, reduce or discriminate relationships in which divergences between the partners may have serious consequences. In this way, drug users do not expose themselves to the need to dissimulate their behaviour. This result can be all the more easily achieved when drug users live alone.

Drug use scenarios

Presentation

In this section, we try to describe the modalities of the relationship between users and drugs, considering what we call drug use scenarios. These result from a combination of several dimensions that, in a more or less pronounced way, according to the trajectories, contribute to characterising the individuals' drug use experiences.

Two dimensions seem to us in the first instance to be defining ones: 1) on the one hand, the degree of autonomy that individuals claim to have over drug use decisions, which can be aligned on an axis that takes, at one pole, a situation of addictive use (at least in relation to some of the drugs used) and, at the other pole, a situation in which consumption is considered optional, that is it can take place or not according to the individuals' decisions; 2) we then considered the locus of consumption, distinguishing on the one hand a private space, delimited in essence by possible proximity relations within a primary group and, on the other hand, a public space where consumption is motivated in essence by circumstances or opportunities exogenous to individuals, involving others who may not be close by and spaces that are not habitual ones in the individuals' lives.

As is evident, the polarisation of these dimensions corresponds only to limiting figures that indicate positions and does not exhaust the variety of the empirical situations observed — in the first place because these empirical situations, in the expression of the individual drug users that we are interested in capturing here, rarely allow themselves to be captured in abrupt and unequivocal representations. Feelings of "addiction" (on the axis of autonomy in relation to the decision to consume) or of exclusion (as a possible figure of a locus of consumption) may be dominant at certain moments of the interview, but denied at others, when the aim is to highlight the capacity of control that one "still" has over consumption. In fact, in many of the biographies analysed, multiple drug use (for example, the use of two substances in the same period) makes it difficult to know which substances weighs more heavily in the need to continue using. Moreover, depending on the representation that individuals have of their situation, discourses may be oriented more on one side than on the other of the vectors considered and the very contents of the vectors may be changed; this means that evaluation of the "control" of consumption or its "consequences" must in this type of analysis be considered based on the subjectivity of individuals. Secondly, we must stress that, besides the fact that the markers of a position may oscillate throughout the interview, the consumption itineraries of the same individual may indeed take in different positions, as we shall see below.

To the two main dimensions we have just presented—the degree of autonomy in relation to the decision to consume and the locus of consumption—we can add two others that allow us to better clarify the orientations produced: 1) on the one hand, the types of substances consumed, since several substances can be opposed to each other, with the most striking representation opposing the use of heroin to that of all other substances, as one to be avoided; 2) on the other hand, self-identity, that is, the totalisation that individuals make of their lives, which in limiting cases distinguishes those who consider their lives to be dominated by consumption from those who tend to play down the importance and meaning of consumption in their lives, taking the view that they do not cease to be who they are because they consume and that their will prevails over their consumption.

In the figure below we represent the modal positions that mark the drug use scenarios resulting from the combination of these four dimensions or vectors and which we shall briefly present below[22].

[22] Although we recognise the interest represented by knowledge of the relations with consumption and substances, we shall limit the analysis here to what is strictly necessary to be able to frame relations with secrecy and the dissimulation practices, which constitute the central object of this note.

Figure 2-1. Drug use scenarios

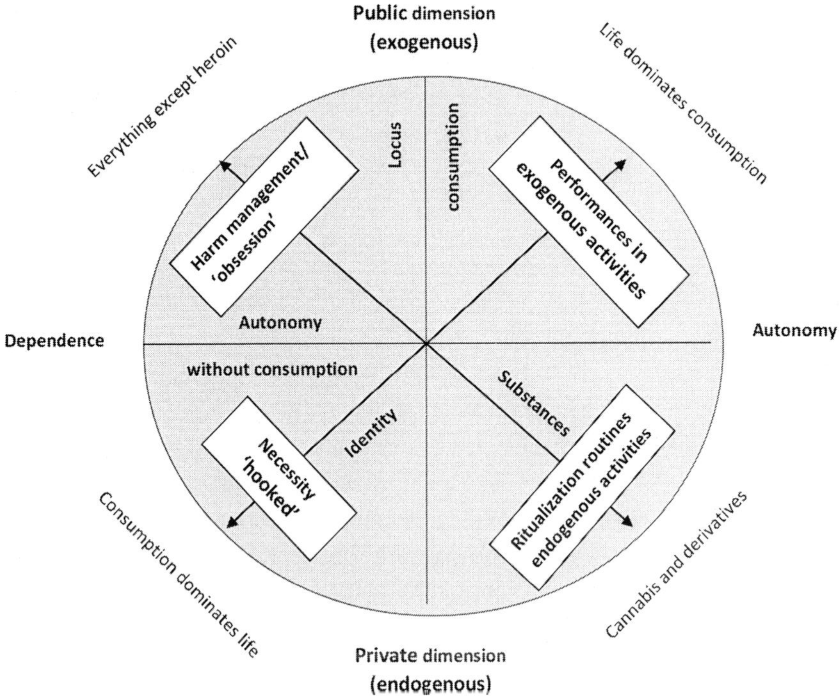

The dependence scenario represents the culmination of a process of disaffiliation (cf. Castel 1995) that jeopardises, at different levels, the usual sociability relationships, which may be limited, according to the substances consumed and the consumption styles, to the strict core of the consumption group or close relatives, when family relationships endure. Social integration can take place, at the limit, at a level of social exclusion or in spaces of exclusion (Balsa 2006). Individuals feel that their lives are controlled by consumption.

Various types of biography may fit the scenario where the dominant concern is with managing the damage associated with consumption, from phases of abstinence in treatment processes to the integration of dependence into lifestyles, especially when it comes to professional activities linked or connoted with consumption. In any of these circumstances, the concern is to control the effects of the substances (to "domesticate" them), particularly in the case of heroin. In cases where consumption is suspended, there is also the concern of not succumbing to the routines associated with previous consumption (particularly spaces and sociability groups).

Scenarios of performative consumption in exogenous activities appear associated with activities or occasions that are considered to require performances in situations or contexts understood as non-routine. Consumption is concentrated on those occasions or for those activities and usually does not interfere or is not part of the individuals' the daily routines: rather, these are extraordinary activities or festive occasions that have their own rhythms and whose initiative is usually exogenous. The substances consumed are generally chosen for the purposes of performance and contact.

Finally, in the scenarios of ritual use, essentially dominated by cannabis and its derivatives, consumption is integrated into the habitual routines of individuals. The ritual dimension—the choice of the moment, activity or occasion—seems to be important in these situations, constituting above all a way of signalling a lifestyle where "smoking a joint" marks a difference. It is a lifestyle that can be passed on, through appropriate socialisation, to members of the household or other relatives and can be shared with close friends who are able to understand them. Sometimes this type of consumption is preceded by the use of other substances, in some cases with a history of dependence.

Below, we shall proceed to a more detailed description of each of these scenarios, considering some dimensions that seem to us to be most significant from the point of view of dissimulation: 1) the substances consumed and the consumption profile; 2) personal identity and its relation with control over consumption; 3) the relational dimension; 4) the socio-affective dimension; 5) the relation with values; and 6) the socio-affective evaluation of the situation. Based on another work where we specifically developed the construction of spaces of transgression (Balsa 2021) we have included in this list the analysis of the spatial dimensions of the dissimulation of consumption, which we shall take up again later.

In Table 2-1 we try to synthesise the modal orientations of each scenario, based on the selected dimensions.

Table 2-1. Modal orientations of consumption scenarios

Dimensions	C1 Addiction	C2 Recent emergence from dependence	C3 Performative consumption	C4 Ritual consumption
Substances	Heroin Cocaine	“Everything, except heroin”	Ecstasy Acid Cocaine	Hashish
Relation with control	Uncontrolled consumption	(On way to) abstinence or assisted consumption	Occasional/periodic consumption	Consumption integrated in life routines
Personal identity	Situation of disaffiliation or feeling of betraying trust of significant others	Difficult interaction with others	“It’s all in the head of each person”	Self-esteem, search for a “state of mind” or “lifestyle”
Relational dimension	Consumption solitary or in support groups / “There are no friends in drugs”	Attempt to recover lost social relations, excluding those associated with consumption	Consumption is relational / Festive, evasive (of one self) or performative	Consumption in family or affective groups / A secret that is shared
Relation with values	Decay of values, doing what one could never have expected to do	In search of lost values, despite others	Neither what the “government wants”, nor what the will dictates	Within values, but with a more open mind
Evaluation of situation	“Hell on Earth”	Heaven is not necessarily guaranteed when you aim to stop consumption	Situation of tension that you need to know how to manage	Valuing of proximity relations/Socialisation of children: “Better to consume at home than in the street”
Relation with space	Confined spaces / “spaces of exclusion”	Support spaces / Spaces compatible with the life that is desired and the life that is rejected	Spaces of leisure or escape / Spaces for interaction with people that may be distant	Dwelling / Spaces of interaction with people who are close

Dependence scenarios: an exile from life

Polyconsumption experiences and the prevalence of certain substances over time are common to most of the biographies we collected. However, the situations of dependence that we now analyse always include the use of heroin or cocaine and, in some cases, both. Although the addictive effects of other substances are emphasised, heroin is considered to occupy a special place. The *"vicious circle"* of consumption (E4/R53) means that *"individuals on heroin, the only thing they think about is heroin, there's nothing else"* (E8/R81). In all the cases analysed here consumption is considered a necessity ("to avoid withdrawal") and is evaluated negatively [*"Coke is already like a punishment that I impose on myself"* (E5/R175)].

The representation of heroin as a "strong" drug that is stigmatised as such, beyond the actual technologies of ingestion, may at the outset justify that its use requires spaces hidden away from the gaze of strangers. However, this condition, which applies to any other illicit substance, albeit in more attenuated fashion, is compatible with any space, taking into account the circumstances and meanings associated with different phases of heroin use.

It thus seems to us that besides considering the spaces where consumption takes place, which exhaust in their physical or functional configurations the spatial meanings of consumption, we must mobilise other dimensions that are important to model the places conducive to consumption, particularly when, as in the case that concerns us here, it is compulsive. In this sense, we know that the progression of consumption towards dependence tends to reduce relationships and therefore to restrict the spaces not only of consumption but also of habitation. Firstly, the relationship with non-drug users is affected. Then, the progression of consumption also leads to a reduction in friends who consume, at the same time as the interests associated with meeting up also begin to be limited to consumption, which finally becomes a solitary activity. Even the space of the house may be restricted, and relationships limited according to the needs of consumption: *"My boyfriend spent weeks and weeks shut up inside the flat, with a scorching sun outside, but with him shut up, in the dark, and injecting himself"* (E4/R53).

We must, however, distinguish situations according to the resources of the drug users. Despite sharing common characteristics, experiences of consumption may vary, depending for example on the stage at which people are in a process of disaffiliation; these stages undoubtedly have variable geometries and combine with the effects of social origin itself.

Consumption restricted to the solitude of the "house" or "room" is contrasted to what happens on the "street" — two opposite ways of experiencing drug dependence that nevertheless include intermediate positions.

In the case of "street" addicts, solitary drug use represents less a whim than the need for protection in spaces where consumption and trafficking bring together people who *"if they had to sell their soul to the devil for some juice, they would do it."* (E11/R45) In this world *"a person using drugs can't be friends with anyone!"* (E11/R26).

The alternative to these spaces that bring together trafficking and use may be the mattress that one of our interviewees occupies in an old factory where she lives and where the interview took place. She has already been through treatment, she has already been "clean", but she ended up going back to consuming. The "road" is the other space she frequents, to prostitute herself, with its being understood that the need to consume justifies any means. Transgression is, in these cases, clearly acknowledged: *"In this world there are no friends, no values, nothing, anything goes."* (E11/R45, E18/R166).

This descent into hell [*"This is hell on Earth"* (E23/R78)] is not observed in the case of addicts who manage to maintain sources of income without needing to transgress. However, it does not take that much for addictive use to be considered a transgression of moral codes when, for example, relationships of trust or compassion are at stake. One of the interviewees will give up using of heroin (while continuing, sporadically, to use other drugs) because she considers that she cannot keep lying to her parents (another of whose children died of an overdose): *"I stopped using on my own initiative so they would never know"* (E1/R59). Transgression can also be read in relation to a valued personal and social identity: *"If you have some respect for yourself..."* (E23/R78).

The boundary between the inside and the outside, which is experienced dramatically in the opposition between "street" and "house" and the bosom of the family to which it generally corresponds may thus also be observed within the household itself, when consumption, whether dissimulated or not, forces a segmentation of the common space. This boundary may also be porous when addicted users continue to benefit from family support.

Finally, let us consider a type of space established for consumption, associated with the situation of addictive use. These, as already mentioned, are spaces where it is possible to sell and use drugs and that benefit from some degree of tolerance on the part of the instances of control (we exclude medically supported spaces that, we reiterate, do not interest us here). Some of these spaces, whose functions are known even outside user groups [*"Everybody knows (laughs)"* (E1/R58)], are mentioned in the biographies we collected, sometimes because they were frequented at some point in individuals' consumption career. Although they may be frequented by buyers from different social backgrounds, these spaces concentrate resident and occasional users, some with profiles of extreme disaffiliation. Connoted as spaces of exclusion, their physical delimitation, which is sometimes well marked, is reinforced by the fact that they are located in areas considered to be unadvisable and dangerous, so that frequenting them requires precautions and minimal socialisation. These spaces of consumption are thus physically delimited, publicly recognised for their functions, and represented as having their own properties that distinguish them from neighbouring spaces. Furthermore, they offer resources that make them attractive to certain drug users *"who like the scene"* (E1/R54) and identify with it, thus constituting *"a scene that becomes addictive"* (Ibidem).

Scenarios of emergence from dependence: the difficult recovery of a "paradise" (or perhaps not) lost

The analysis of scenarios of "coming out of addiction" allows us to complement our understanding of scenarios of "addiction" but also to understand the relationships that exist between them. In the cases looked at above, the substance at the origin of the dependence was heroin, sometimes associated with cocaine. For that reason, one of the marks that characterises well this scenario at the level of narratives is the desire to move away from the circumstances associated with consumption, and the radical rejection of heroin: *"Anything but heroin"* (E8/E15/E27/E32). The decision to quit heroin and suspend the situation of dependence does not always imply giving up the use of other substances. The scenarios of quitting are not necessarily the last in the consumption stories entrusted to us, because periods of quitting can be followed by periods of relapse.

At the level of individual identities and the relationship with control, the decision to stop consuming may depend on multiple factors whose importance seems to us to be above all associated with the idiosyncrasies of the individual stories.

At the moral level, if the desire to respect certain values (for example, the feeling of compassion and the desire not to betray the trust of people who are close) can influence the decision to stop consuming, the failure to respect these values by those who are considered to be able to help (for example, the people who are closest, or representatives of institutions) can, on the contrary, hinder it.

Since addictive use is associated with life routines and certain spaces, one of the conditions considered to be decisive for quitting is to break with these routines, for example no longer frequenting the spaces and friends with whom one used to consume.

The assessment of the situations that fit with the scenario of constrained use are, as we saw above, negative: *"hell on Earth"* in the words of one interviewee. However, the decision to quit does not by itself, nor in a linear way, make it possible to "go to heaven": *"And I go where? That's the problem!"* (E11/R73). The outcome of decisions appears to be very dependent on consumption histories and on the capacity that drug users have to mobilise resources, which do not depend exclusively on the social class of origin, since there are situations in which social resources exist but are annulled by the punishment exercised by families on the basis of moral codes, and others in which the continued support from family facilitates quitting in disadvantaged social environments.

"Home" is undoubtedly an important resource when stopping consuming, but its viability is not always guaranteed. Several types of situations may occur. There are those in which home was never absent, so that winning it back only requires the re-establishment of a moral order and an ethic of relationships compatible with the loyalty and respect that people think is owed to close relatives. While this moral order is not restored with the end of consumption, the figure of "hell" that serves to characterise consumption contexts, moves into the home itself [*"Nowadays there are big troubles at home"* (E15/R124)]. The fact that the family home remains open, after being abandoned, facilitates the reorientation, in synergy with any recourse to institutions of treatment. However, the return to a family home that has been abandoned can pose multiple obstacles due to the loss of trust, particularly when there are successive attempts at quitting, or to the dismantling of the original family unit, for instance after the end of conjugal relationships or the removal of parental rights. It can also happen that the home that was abandoned is seen as a possible support but is closed off forever. The relationship with the "home" as an object to be won back allows us to better understand the negative meanings attributed to the spaces of addictive use, especially when the figure of the "home" is invoked in the broadest sense of protection.

This means that the spaces related to the processes of stopping addictive use appear to have to be constructed, in the same way as the spaces for consumption, considering the various levels of determinations that weigh in people's lives. Under these circumstances, policies relating to institutional treatment and reintegration in society, which fall outside the scope of this work, may offer alternative places to those that consumption has destroyed forever.

Scenarios of management of consumption risks in festive or performative settings: construction of places of exception

This scenario is associated with the idea that consumption is a way to have experiences outside those associated with banal everyday life. In one of the variants we observed, the use of acid[23] constitutes a divergence from "reality", making possible an opening up to new dimensions of personal identities. With the use of ecstasy or acid, one experiences *"your body speeding up"* (E17/R175), a greater relational capacity [*"I get much more sociable, talking to people"* (E17/R79)], or all this at the same time. But the same effect of exceptionality in relation to everyday life [*"You're unlikely to relate so well with people without using ecstasy or LSD"* (E19/R58)] is

[23] These classifications are approximate, and it is not appropriate here to distinguish the many varieties, cuts or degrees of purity of the different types of substance, which can therefore produce different effects.

also obtained with cocaine use, when the target is relational or professional performances that mobilise self-esteem and stimulate certain individual skills.

Despite their diversity, the types of consumption that we consider in this scenario share the fact that they are represented as occurring in a circumstantial way; that is, even if they take place periodically, they are associated with events or situations outside the usual frameworks of everyday life. This, however, does not prevent the use of these substances from being frequent and intensive, nor stop individuals from regularly (sometimes daily) using cannabis or one of its derivatives, even if one excludes the possibility of these consumptions arising from situations of dependence that are not, however, acknowledged by the individuals, who, on the contrary, argue for a position of autonomy in relation to consumption.

Thus, by focusing this scenario on "risk management" strategies, we cannot assume that they in all circumstances actually result in controlled use. Regardless of these levels of control (which, incidentally, we could never verify with our means of observation), risk management strategies are defined by drug users themselves, who cite them as the way they relate to substances. The principle of this management is formulated by one of the interviewees, who considers that, on the one hand, *"drugs can't be seen as the government wants them to be seen"* but, on the other, neither can they be treated *"as the human being tends to treat them: since it's there, you can abuse it at will"*... Refusing both extremes (*"it has nothing to do with that"*), the solution would be for consumption to be accepted as having *"a purpose, not to be an addiction, but to cause liberation of the mind, to allow altered states of consciousness"* (E19/R36). It is clear that this openness to the strategy can be manifested with varying degrees of conviction, from those who seek to affirm their total autonomy in relation to the decision to consume to those who seem only to want to get away from a situation that presents as much less under control than they give to understand.

The control that one believes one has over this type of consumption may be associated with different dimensions. The responsibility due to the consumer to not allow a consumption "habit" to turn into an "addiction" can be placed, first of all, on the person themselves, on their "willpower". This willpower may involve defining a discipline deemed appropriate for managing risks, such as setting targets or consumption rules. This self-control may also be assumed at the level of the group. Another dimension associated with the capacity of control is the actual culture of drugs use in question — the sporadic use of ecstasy, acid and cocaine, because it are considered occasional and, as opposed to heroin, permit of being modulated.

In this scenario, drug use is rarely solitary. It is mainly associated with socialising, often in festive environments, with sharing in a group being important, and substances considered as "engines" or aides to physical, psychological or relational performance.

The consumption spaces involved in this scenario may be very varied, considering the distinct cultures and subcultures of consumption. Raves, trances or other performative consumption situations that obey certain canons that regulate their modes of organisation, the way they take place, or their duration require appropriate spaces that may vary greatly. This means that, in this type of scenario, the need to construct a place of consumption overlaps with the very space that is used.

Thus, in this type of drug use, spaces may be pondered from multiple perspectives, such as, for example: 1) being "closed" or "open" [*"Normally trance parties are always in the middle of nowhere"* (E20/R313)]; 2) being organised or not by some instance external to the individuals [the "system", where *"there are many people who go there to cause trouble"* against "nature" and where "[you feel] free" (E20/R327)]; 3) being connoted with the night or with the day [*"This... because it appears really linked to working at night...and going out at night"* (E2/R79)]; 4) their being work or leisure spaces, or at least ones that are not constrained by professional commitments [*"more going out than working"* (E2/R79)]; 5) their being spaces where one usually consumes or other spaces [*"If I'd stayed there, I don't know if I would have held myself back or not... coming [here] in that sense... was beneficial, because it made me use over a much longer period of time, you know?"* (E6/R25)]; 6) they allow the act of consumption to be hidden, especially when it requires some ritual, such as the preparation of a line of cocaine, for example [*"In the bar, you don't get something out and make a line there and sniff it, right? Everyone's watching! Just like I don't go to the bathroom and sniff! I don't feel good about going to a bathroom to have a sniff... it's like, you leave the disco, get into a car... If there's not much, I even do it inside the car, it's my property, that's what the law says."* (E33/R136)].

We may say, resorting to a formula often used by Jean Remy, that these different dimensions constitute a matrix from which the meanings of the individual positions are constructed, according to a variable geometry. What makes a great variety of spaces meaningful from the perspective of consumption is the way of marking them with elements that make them moments of exception that are sought to be created through consumption. This marking may be suggested through artefacts (decoration, light effects, colours, type of music, sound volume...) or elements invested with particular meanings (such as nature...), creating settings suitable for each of the subcultures one wishes to promote [*"Those parties or raves that are especially worth it for the music or the space. Okay, it has to have a set of factors to be worth it, to be able to say it's a party, right?"* (E30/R153)] and which can be reproduced in any space. The recognition of these conditions creates expectations that become sedimented with use, giving rise to emblematic places for such a type of consumption. However, on the one hand, *"there are people who are there and don't consume"* (E1/R70) and, on the other, *"there are people who just because they don't have a tablet or acid don't go to the party. That's not OK... The important thing isn't having something to take or not, the important thing is to like trance... It's OK for me to go there and take something or not."* (E20/R326) But then, if one can participate without using, beyond the staging that predisposes to consumption what is that truly leads people to do so? Probably a need to appropriate the staged space to produce their own place. The staged space is not sufficient for different reasons: 1) on the one hand, some of its elements can be reproduced in other spaces: *"Cafés, nightclubs, bars, parties and all that"* (E32/R47); *"I hear the sound the same as I hear the sound here at home, or in the café"* (E20/R327); 2) on the other hand, the very conditions of these spaces may be difficult to bear [*"Okay, it's possible [not to consume] up to a certain point, because it's almost impossible to be there at that thing"* (E20/R327)]; 3) finally, with time, the effects of staging become banal [*"Also with age and the actual interest of the thing... It started to become such a routine thing that it lost its fun, didn't it? So, like that [using], it becomes much more fun."* (E30/R197)].

Besides the effects of staging, these spaces take on specific meanings when they are invested by individuals under the influence of drugs: *"That is like being in a place like any other [but] from the moment you've already taken something it starts that scene of 'it's all beautiful, it's all very beautiful, everything is very beautiful,' because people dress up for the party, everything is very fluorescent, you smile at people, if you bump into someone you apologise..."* (E30/R217) But, when the effects of the staging and its appropriation end, the exceptionality of the spaces and of existence vanishes: *"Then, in the morning, when it's over, then everything isn't beautiful any more; I mean, the party is nice, the people are nice, they dress the same way, I smile, I'm nice and whatever, but at the level of that warmth... you've moved on... You're lucid, you're normal, aren't you? It can't have the same meaning any more."* (E30/R219-220).

Scenarios of ritualised use of cannabis: construction of places integrated in daily life, aimed at achieving states of mind or at maintaining a valued lifestyle

The scenario of ritualised cannabis use shares with the previous scenario a controlled representation of consumption, on thc axis of autonomy, but opposes it on the axis of the loci of consumption. In the scenario of the management of occasional use the privileged spaces are public, whereas in the ritualised use of cannabis the consumptions are more in conjunction with private spaces. Cannabis (and all its derivatives) is, at this scenario, the only substance consumed, even though other substances may have been consumed previously. Furthermore, we do not consider here situations in which cannabis is consumed regularly, but in a secondary way and sometimes as an adjunct to other substances. Also excluded are situations of consumption recognised by the drug users themselves as being 'harmful'.

Contrary to the previous scenario, in which consumption was carefully separated from daily life, at moments of exception, typical users in scenarios of ritualised cannabis use are distinguished by integrating moments of rupture in their daily life routines: *"It's a life option"* (E4/R71); *"It's a way of being, it's the search for [a] state of mind."* (E4/R67).

Rather than being associated with specific goals, consumption is part of life routines (at weekends or to make love, for example), which can be daily, in the form of rituals of decompression or transition. However, they can also be facilitators of certain daily tasks: *"A bit like a spring"* (E4/R6), or to resolve some "anxieties". But the most significant expressions of this scenario are produced in conjunction with the family setting and with sociabilities at the level of social groups, making it possible better to portray some of their modal orientations.

The family level coincides, as a rule, with the domestic space, although it may on certain occasions include other family members who do not belong to the household. Consumption that takes place in the domestic space at first constitutes, in opposition to the external space, moments of decompression in the face of stress or tiredness. The demarcation between domestic and work spaces is particularly clear, but the distinction between rest and activity can also be made within the domestic space itself.

Consumption in a group is more associated with its affective or relational dimension. The transgressive dimension of consumption may bring greater complicity to relationships, like a *"secret that is shared"* (E4/R27, E27/R148). As in the case of domestic consumption, the ritual dimension is also underscored here.

The need to control risks is essentially absent: *"It became a habit, not an addiction"* (E8/R94). This lack of vigilance is often justified by the possibility that consumption is interrupted when the substance is missing. The fact that many of these drug users have experimented with other substances before seems to give them a sense of the measure used in this evaluation, in considering that the effects of a "joint" are much more controllable than those of other substances. This does not mean that certain effects on themselves or on people close to them may not sometimes be questioned. In the main, however, an evaluation in terms of normative conformity of this type of consumption is made: *"With hashish we are still behaving in accordance with the values, our values don't change"* (E4/R50/1).

According to the two modal orientations described—domestic use and recreational use—the spaces of consumption are the home itself (or its extensions, such as holidays or family gatherings) and places of conviviality. As in the previous situation, there may be multiple convivial spaces, so it is a matter of constructing the places deemed most adequate for the rituals to take place according to the desired pattern, allowing consumption with some discretion.

In the domestic variant of cannabis use, the "house" or the "family environment" are represented as places of safe and controlled consumption as opposed to unsafe consumption outside. From this perspective, the home can be a means to socialise young people into "responsible" consumption. When, inside the domestic space, the youngest are not allowed to witness consumption, the construction of the room as a place of consumption may depend on the door of a bedroom being closed.

Conclusions: consumption spaces, places and territories

Starting from two dimensions that seemed to us to clarify the orientations of consumption behaviours—on the one hand, greater or lesser autonomy in relation to the decision to consume and, on the other, the more public or more private orientation of the loci—we were able to construct a typology of positions that we called consumption scenarios.

These scenarios outline only some of the modal orientations in which consumption may take place, and may be associated not only with the basic dimensions that constitute them, but also with certain substances and with the representation that individuals have of themselves as drug users, which, at the limit, separates those who feel that they "live for consumption" from those who consider that their consumption is controlled by their own life choices.

The isolated types that represent consumption orientations do not constitute individual phases, because individuals can move between them at a certain point of their itineraries. Representing modes of relationship with substances, individuals can circulate between each scenario, although certain passages are easier than others. Thus, a ritual user of hashish, in some cases a former consumer of other substances, may if circumstances allow use another recreational substance, usually excluding heroin. In the scenario of performative use, the habitual use of hashish is frequent. This consumption, usually associated with occasional events or episodes, is associated with addictive use (to an extent that the limits of our information do not allow us to determine) or is practised by people who have already been addicted. In the scenarios into which where former addicts fit best, we can find individuals who have decided to exclude heroin use, sometimes associated with cocaine, but who may continue to smoke hashish or any of the performative substances.

As they do not constitute types of consumption that are mutually permeable, the scenarios are not profiled as "phases" of a consumption itinerary. No doubt the dependence scenario represents, as we have already said, the end of a process of disaffiliation, on a consumption itinerary that turned out badly, in the same way that the "coming out of addiction" scenario has meaning in relation to the way that the dependence was experienced. However, the transitions between one scenario and another are not always one-way, nor irreversible.

From the perspective of dissimulation strategies, it seemed appropriate to directly relate the space—a prime instrument for hiding—with the consumption scenarios. At this level we observed that conventional spaces, that is those with socially allocated functions, can be associated with certain consumption scenarios or cultures. However, we also saw that these functionalities can be subverted, transforming certain spaces into places of consumption. In fact, most often a place for consumption can be constructed in any space. This transformation does not, however, take place indiscriminately. Everything depends on the intentionality of the consumer, which is not an isolated manifestation of will but rather part of a culturally informed chain that is anchored in certain circumstances. In these cases, in construction their consumption routines, individuals take advantage of the qualities of the spaces most suited to their cultures, but also mould them to their senses, to accommodate the whims of their idiosyncrasics.

All spaces offer a greater or lesser plasticity, depending on the modes of appropriation to which they may be subjected in the process of constructing places of consumption. In turn, there are places in which different spaces may coexist. A closed bedroom door may separate a space of consumption from a space where consumption is excluded. In the space of an abandoned industrial area, where a place of leisure has been constructed suitable for a certain consumer culture, different types of spatialities may coexist, depending for example on whether those who frequent them do or do not use drugs. This leisure space may, at the same time, be a space where a profession is exercised. We shall return later to this versatility of spaces with regard to consumption.

Relation with secrecy and dissimulation in the construction of social relations of consumption

Now we know better the circumstances in which consumption takes place, we can focus on the relationship with secrecy and dissimulation practices. We grant that the publicising of consumption may not have the same importance or the same meaning according to the normative references or the consumption scenarios in relation to which individuals position themselves. We understand, for example, that the need to hide does not arise in the same way when the principle of abstinence is accepted (when the referentials of conformity, dissonance or diffraction are adopted) or, in the opposite direction, when someone consumes arguing for a counter-normative position or a situation of anomie. The different consumption scenarios outline, in the same way, specific zones where confidentiality and secrecy are posed in very distinct ways.

We do not intend to draw this chart in detail, as this would represent an excessive exercise for the goals that we have defined here. Neither do we intend to formulate the relations between dissimulation, normative references and consumption scenarios from a causal point of view, which would open the analysis to a type of approach of an explanatory nature that the type of material we are working with does not make it possible to take. However, moving away from the causal model does not exempt us from considering the ways in which the different variables are related that intervene in the definition of the positions adopted by individuals. How, then, are individual biographies, normative references and the scenarios in which consumption takes place related in the definition of strategies of dissimulation?

Moving away from causal reasoning, we seek to answer these questions by adopting a comprehensive approach of the actancial type that presupposes, as Jean-Michel Berthelot (Berthelot 1998) has clearly defined it, a set of actors and a set of actions interacting in a common social space on the basis of which, according to the always specific circumstances of each situation, individuals decide their strategies and, based on the question in which we are interested here, their strategies of dissimulation of behaviour. This scheme of actantial intelligibility no doubt corresponds best to the space of analysis that Jean Remy connotes with the problematic of the social transaction (Remy 2005, 2015; Remy, Voyé and Servais 1978) that we have developed in another paper[24].

In this sense, the relation with secrecy and the practices of dissimulation perceived on the basis of individual practices will be considered as analysing elements. This means that, instead of from the outset keeping our understanding of individual practices within a mould of *a priori* causality, we prefer to consider that the conditions of publicising and the rules of confidentiality through which individuals view their consumption, reacting to the idiosyncrasies of individual biographies, clarify their positions in relation to different normative frameworks while at the same time making possible a better understanding of the consumption scenarios in which they position themselves.

The approach we propose to the social relations of drug use, from the perspective of dissimulation, involves first analysing the ways in which individuals conceal their use. We shall then consider practices of dissimulation in various contexts that seem most relevant to us, distinguishing: 1) relations in formal situations (usually institutional environments) and 2) proximity relations, within which we can also differentiate friendship relations and family relations.

A semantic space of secrecy

But, after all, how can one hide? How can the theoretical orientations we discussed above be updated do we updated in the case of illicit substance use? Before analysing the circumstances in which concealment takes place, the information we have collected allows us to understand that the practices of "hiding" or "not hiding" may result from different semantic fields that allow concealment to take on different meanings, including from the perspective of ethical or affective commitments that individuals have in relation to those from whom they hide.

---

[24] Cf. "A construção de espaços de transgressão: o consumo de drogas", in *Cidades, Escalas e Transações*, Col. Navegar é Preciso. Vila Nova de Famalicão: Húmus, 2021.

a) Dissipating by showing

In the manner of Edgar Allan Poe's trick in the short story "The Purloined Letter" (in Portuguese, "A Carta Roubada", Poe 2011), one possible way to hide consumption is to do it in plain sight, i.e. in places where one does not expect to be able to hide something [*"With time I came to learn that the more hidden away the place is, the more of a show you put on."* (E6/R25)] It is thus a matter of showing in order to better hide. Indeed, to show, while thinking that one is hiding, exposes the consumer to the risk that someone, an improbable character in the imagined scene, really sees what was supposed not to be seen: *"Here [city] I am very comfortable and sometimes people pass by who shouldn't see and who will tell my mother. Many people know me, and I don't know them."* (E17/R260) That is, the anonymity sought in dissipation cannot be decided unilaterally, since the individual does not eliminate another who wants to see, nor the density of a social relation that even anonymity constitutes.

b) Pretending: the world of make believe

This relational density also allows makes it possible to explain the position of those who see and know, without wanting to: *"Even though they [the parents] know, I had to tell them."* (E32/R112) In these circumstances the secret is a factor in both directions in the relationship: *"Yes [they hide it from their friend], but I think it is that thing of I know that you know that I know! It's just that it's better not to even touch on that subject."* (E23/R91) Or pretending that one does not know, for the time being: *"My relationship with my parents then started to get worse, too, and they also started to suspect... My mother was very suspicious and I think she even knew... she really knew, but she didn't take it very seriously"* (E29/R130).

c) Lying, firstly to oneself

Another construction, which may in some cases feed a form of illusion, allows occasional consumption (activities, meetings, celebrations, etc.) to be hidden even from the consumer. Once it is considered to be under control, consumption is dressed up in a way that tends to attenuate, or even deny, its importance. One of the ways of doing this is to exacerbate the level of control that one has over consumption: *"I want to and I can are the only two big reasons why I do it."* (E6/R83) The importance of consumption can also be denied based on: 1) the place that it has in the consumer's life [*"It is important, but it's an importance like this [gesture showing it as small]; it's like me enjoying going to the beach because it is sunny; from time to time I like to smoke cocaine because I feel good, I don't get richer, poorer, fatter, thinner, it doesn't influence me at all"* (E6/R114); *"But then, okay, we're talking about using, but I don't use drugs anyway, I don't turn drugs into daily use or anything. I take it as a bit of fun"* (E3/R38)]; 2) its frequency [*"It's never more than twice a month, I can assure you of that"* (E6/R78)]; 3) or the effects it has [*"It's not [serious], it's the same as drinking a beer. In fact, it's been proven that smoking a joint is less harmful than smoking a cigarette, you know? Drinking a coffee is worse than smoking a joint, so, this is scientific data, it's just that socially and culturally people don't assimilate this"* (E6/R61)]. Finally, the potential risk or the "infraction" of using can also be played down: *"There are a lot of people, you know? In fact, if you knew the amount of people and the positions that these people have here who use drugs, you'd be amazed. Here, in the government, anywhere, everywhere there are people that do... Drugs are in everything, in the government, in parliament, in medicine, in everything, and that's an accepted fact, you know?"* (E6/R61).

This repackaging justifies a type of occasional and controlled use, although as in Hans Christian Andersen's tale there may be a moment when it becomes clear that "the emperor has no clothes". Some of the itineraries we analysed make it possible to understand that the frequency of consumption may not respect the desire to control them: *"At the beginning when I started experimenting, it was at the weekend, once in a while, once a month at the most. Sometimes a long time would go by without my even thinking about it... But then it started to become more frequent... first it was one weekend a month, then it was two, then it was three, then it was four... then it was Friday and Saturday, then it was Friday, Saturday and Sunday... then it was during the week, then it was Monday, Tuesday and Wednesday and then it became one day after another... and it was all a very gradual evolution. Things went on and on and on... until you found yourself completely addicted, both psychologically and physically."* (E1/R41)

d) Hiding by turning away from others' gaze

The most commonly mentioned types of concealment, however, are those that seek to keep consumption away from any gaze, especially indiscreet ones. This may involve hiding moments of consumption or not showing oneself in compromising places or situations. As it will become clear below, it is not a matter of keeping only moments of consumption away from the gaze of others, but also any mark that may give it away, namely its physical or psychological effects.

e) Eliminating evidence

Erasing signs that could give away consumption is thus another of the modalities of concealment: *"I wasn't very visible... I always tried to take care of myself as much as possible, so that no one would be suspicious. It's not like certain people who really let themselves go and are all sloppy, unshaven, with uncut hair..."* (E28/R94); *"Even if I come home very drunk, I always end up disguising it. I don't know if they notice or not, at least they've never said anything to me."* (E36/R94) This type of dissimulation is easier to manage when the effects of consumption can be hidden: *"When I'm going to do it, it's something that can last from six to nine hours, or twelve hours that you can be under the influence... Normally when you do it, you already know that the next day you have to be free... Since you already know that, you do things in such a way that the next day you can rest"* (E9/R217); *"There are things that, after I do them, I don't even show up in front of my parents: if I go to a party I spend two days away from home, I come home the day after, or two days after, when I'm healthy and have had a bath."* (E32/R125) This strategy can also involve not leaving traces *"Although my parents don't go through my things a lot, I don't walk around with things on show"* (E36/R94); *"I was very stupid, too. I would leave everything there in my room, you see, I would hide everything but very badly. And my mother, well, she would go there and... my mother would find silver foil and I don't know what else..."* (E28/R68). In the same way, one can "clean up" one's body before going to the doctor. Since the signs of consumption can indeed be very varied, this means that the strategies followed to hide them are also very varied: *"As I don't... I don't inject, they'd never realise that way, right? I don't need to cover my arms or anything like that"* (E37/R72).

f) Separating routines or contexts, or selecting relationships

But concealment can result from the simple fact that the times and spaces of consumption do not coincide with those that are shared with the people from whom one wants to hide: *"When I get home after a night out, they're sleeping, aren't they? They end up never seeing me."* (E36/R94) At the limit, hiding becomes easier when the contexts of life are separate: *"As I live alone, most of the time I don't have to hide anything."* (E1/R66) But one can also hide by selecting the people with whom one socialises: *"I try to hang out with people who don't have that kind of prejudice."* (E7/R62)

g) Lying by denying the truth

Lying is the modality that makes it possible to hide when confronted by someone who cannot know, according to the geography that is designed for secrecy. But lying can take different forms.

First of all, one can lie by denying the truth: *"My parents tried to get it all out of me, but I [would say] — 'I don't, I don't get mixed up in that, I don't get mixed up in that'. I always tried to hide it as much as possible, until one day..."* (E28/R257); *"I've been confronted by my mother: she told me to my face that I smoked hashish and I said no. I try to deny it, whenever I can."* (E17/R258).

h) Lying by deceiving with the truth

One can lie by deceiving, using the truth: *"I always say no, I mean, I always let them think, I didn't deny it directly, but I always let them think that I had never used drugs... But if they knew, it wouldn't be such a terrible thing. If sometimes it comes up in conversation how much drugs there are [when you go out] at night and whatever, and I say 'I know that, I know that, I work at night and I see how things are'; it is just an effort at containment."* (E2/R112).

i) Lying by not telling the whole truth

One also lies when one does not tell the whole truth: *"Yes, my work colleagues, not least since I am working in that setting, whether on the magazine or at the production company, it's a more or less normal thing that people know that I use, not all drugs, of course, but at least hashish, and sometimes LSD or ecstasy, they know. In relation to cocaine that is something that, as it happens, I ... it's not something that I like to say I consume"* (E32/R118); *"They [parents] never knew about the acid, it was always just the 'puffs'."* (E7/R139).

These different figures take shape through the different dimensions associated with the practices of dissimulation, which we shall detail below. We consider first the situations of dissimulation that occur in formal circumstances or spaces and then move on to analyse the construction of dissimulation relations in situations of sociability of proximity.

Construction of social relations of dissimulation

The social relations of concealment are motivated, in the first instance, by the referential of abstinence, in its imperative dimension, even before the specific protocols that concretise them in practice are considered, taking into account the normative referential and the consumption scenarios that frame each particular consumption situation. Thus, hiding is not a whim of individuals to singularise themselves: one hides because, according to the social codes agreed upon, one should not show oneself because that would imply harmful consequences, both for the one who hides and for the one from whom something is hidden. However, while the referential of abstinence clearly sets the boundary between what may and may not be shown, it does not provide guidelines on how one may hide, insofar as this would mean acknowledging the existence of the behaviour that is, from the outset, proscribed. This also means that, faced with a consumption situation, individual drug users are faced with the need to invent modalities and strategies through which, depending on the circumstances, they will hide, allow to be seen, or show.

Taking into account the greater or lesser probability of socio-affective involvement of individuals in relationships, we shall structure the analysis by considering, firstly, the relationships developed in more formal contexts, dominated by functional relations, and then the relationships that are developed in situations of socio-affective proximity.

Hiding in formal contexts

By formal contexts, we shall consider those that may be more connoted, at the outset, with institutions that have responsibilities in defining normative frameworks of abstinence or that are mandated to defend them: the forces of law and order, in defence of the legal norm, and doctors, in defence of the health norm, represent two institutions responsible for defending the ideal of abstinence (notwithstanding all the inflections that this principle may suffer, as mentioned above). The Church may also be mobilised as the defender of a moral order. We shall also take into account work contexts where, despite the controversies they may give rise to with regard to their relationship with consumption[25], considerations of a legal, health and even moral order are involved. Finally, we consider the disposition of individuals to declare their consumption in the situation of a formal interview at home, carried out by a stranger, face to face. This situation interests us particularly, since the answers that we obtain allow us to define the conditions of application of our survey (cf. previous chapter).

Instances of authority and control

Taking situations of communication in a formal context, one can firstly hide by invoking the normative order in force, referring to society as a whole or to some of the institutions that represent it. At this level we observe the impact of censorship exercised by institutions mandated to prevent or punish consumption or to treat its effects.

The police authority represents one of these institutions of vigilance: *"If I'm going to consume with my friends, obviously you should always look out to see if the police are coming or not, what the situation is. You're always a little bit wary, looking to see if you can do it or not."* (E22/R226) When spaces of consumption and also of trafficking are recalled, the appearance of the police or of other less usual characters generates distrust: *"When women, police and men in suits and ties turn up there, they [the dealers] straight away do a double take, because it is really grabs your attention and is not normal there"* (E6/R15).

The public instance, suggested in the figure of the state, seems to prompt a greater distancing: *"At work I think they shouldn't know because these are*

---

[25] Cf. our work on the consumption of alcohol and other drugs by the working population (Balsa, Urbano and Vital 2021).

personal things. And even more when you work in the civil service, for the state, it really affects things a lot." (E30/R245).

Health professionals themselves can be excluded from the circle of confidants: *"I have a family doctor with whom I don't talk about this; I had a psychiatrist with whom I never talked about this"* (E27/R166); *"I've been wanting to go to the doctor for a long time, to have tests and all that, because it's necessary, and I haven't been going because of that. That's why I've been trying to see if I can stop for a month, two months, clean up."* (E19/R165) But consumption is also hidden from professionals potentially associated with treatment for its effects, such as, for example, psychiatrists and psychologists: *"I asked him [my psychiatrist] once if smoking was bad for me and he started laughing... For example, with my psychologist I don't talk about that subject because it doesn't disturb my affectivity and my way of being, of living, my behaviour in relation to the things I want to try to resolve with the psychologist; I don't think there's any reason to talk about it..."* (E4/R118). (E4/R118). The dissimulation of some consumption from the professionals in harm reduction programmes themselves can also be observed: *"In this Centre down there, of the people who take methadone, 90% do drugs, and they take tests and... almost everybody tested positive, and nobody was expelled. Half the people around who use drugs are all from the Centre."* (E25/R152).

Professional context

In addition to being hidden from friends and acquaintances, consumption is also hidden in the workplace: *"My employers, of course, don't know, not because I have a problem with it, but not everyone has the same way of seeing things, there's no point..."* (R10/R150); *"In my job, I certainly wouldn't, I think there are a lot of people who wouldn't understand"* (E4/R135). Even when there is no orientation, in principle, to conceal, consumption is concealed because one is not sure how knowledge of consumption might be understood and what consequences this might have: *"Some [of my colleagues] I wouldn't mind if they knew, but it also doesn't hurt them not knowing... Some of them use [drugs], others have used hashish, but others don't or never have, but they know that I, from time to time, use hashish, cocaine... Every now and then, in conversation, [the subject] came up and I always say no."* (E2/R111)

Formal interview context

The readiness of interviewees to respond to a questionnaire was of particular interest to us from the perspective of the application of the INPG. The interviewees were confronted with the possibility of being asked to respond to such a questionnaire, on the basis that information on consumption would be collected under the responsibility of the University as part of a study of interest to the Ministry of Health, that the interview would take place in the homes of randomly selected people and that responses would be anonymous.

The question was put at the end of the in-depth interview, that is, after all aspects related to consumption had been discussed in detail. Having had no difficulty in discussing this information in front of an interviewer who, although not necessarily known to them, was referred to them by someone who was (the selection of drug users was made using the snowball technique), the individuals were then placed in a situation in which they were asked to talk about their consumption, but now following a completely different interview technique: responding to a questionnaire, applied by an unknown (but duly accredited) interviewer, with the contact being made at their homes.

More than half of the interviewees replied that they would agree to do so, some without reservations, but many with some conditions attached. When presented with this relatively positive response, some interviewers reacted with surprise, rephrasing the question and stressing that it would be a "door-to-door application" with an unknown interviewer... This reaction nevertheless reflects a representation of consumption as a censored (and undoubtedly censorable) behaviour that could not be studied using traditional survey instruments. As one of the interviewees puts it, at the limit, this would be a "violation of confidentiality". On a more positive note, another respondent emphasises the unusual nature of the situation by stating that he refuses to respond to *"interviews like those done by [name of a television channel]"* or through techniques used to find out about other types of consumption: *"If it was a survey about other things, fine... but, well, about hashish..."*. (E29).

In the cases in which the acceptance was without reservations, beyond any availability at that moment, the motivations ranged from an uninhibited *"maybe because I have nothing to hide"* (E14) through an altruistic *"I'm here in this world for some reason. I'd like to send out some message, to talk about the things that are happening to me that could be of help"* (E19); *"Yes, because these initiatives are important and [...] there should be ever more information so that there aren't people talking without knowing [what they're talking about]"* (E28) to an emphatic *"I always answer. I've done loads of interviews of this kind."* (E21).

The negative responses generally denote a defensive and protective attitude on the part of drug users towards a normative framework that they consider to be hostile to them: *"Using drugs is not accepted and people are judged"* (E1); *"I use drugs and it is not well regarded."* (E35) For that reason, *"using drugs isn't something to talk about lightly"* (E1) and, at the limit, asking questions about consumption *"is a bit of a violation of privacy."* (E3) Other situations of refusal are justified by the fear that the suggested conditions of the survey will not be fulfilled [*"That data, whether you like it or not, can sometimes end up in the wrong hands"* (E3)], mainly that of anonymity, due to the fact that the interview is carried out in the household [*"It is very difficult for a person to manage to be completely open with their household behind the door"* (E9)] and that the interviewer is a stranger [*"It's a bit of a delicate subject to talk about with anyone you don't know"* (E35)].

These fears explain why some individuals only agreed to respond to the survey when the conditions that could give them confidence were assured. These conditions are the guarantee of anonymity [*"They could for example introduce that in the censuses, being anonymous"* (E10); *"If you gave me a survey and I closed it so he wouldn't read it... maybe I would be fine to answer it"* (E35)] or at least confidentiality [*"If the degree of confidentiality were guaranteed"* (E2)]. The technique for selecting individuals was a problem for some: *"Door to door, I don't think so. I think I wouldn't feel comfortable answering."* (E1) For others, the issue of confidentiality could be overcome if the conditions allowed for the individual *"to be alone at home"* (E7). For others still, the refusal could be motivated, from the outset, by the distance that the approach implies. Where the interviewer is concerned, there is the fear that they will not have the necessary capacity for empathy: *"It depends on the questions, seeing if it's possible to talk freely... If the person's aim is to comprehend you and understand what you're saying"* (E20). But distance can also result from a lack of trust in those conducting the survey: *"I wouldn't answer, unless the proof was very good, very clear!"* (E2); *"Yes, if it is anonymous and for a national institution, INE [National Statistics Institute], not [name of TV channel]"* (E8).

Dissimulation in social relations of proximity: concealing from whom

We are now interested in understanding how individuals position themselves in relation to secrecy when we consider their involvement in social relations of proximity. We understand relations of proximity as those that are, from the outset, regulated by affective ties even before they become functional ties. This definition includes family and friendship relations. In this sense, relations of proximity may exist in formal contexts, for example, in professional contexts, when functional interests do not imprint their own mark on the relationship. In the same way, we may question the inclusion of family relations in this category, when they exclusively obey functional considerations. We shall see, however, that in this case at least a duty of deference is required.

Friendship relations

Let us consider, firstly, how dissimulation strategies are applied to acquaintances or friends.

A first position will allow us to list the spaces as positioning criteria: *"I don't use drugs here [work city]; I know people here who do, but I don't use with them, I'm not in the habit of doing it here... The people I do it with are people [from city of origin] that I've known for many years..."* (E6/R28). The position is clear and opposes two spaces differentiated by a functional and probably affective relationship: here and there. More than interknowledge and even the proximity with consumption situations (which occur 'here' and 'there'), what is valued is long acquaintance, especially when it seals a good friendship: *"In our group of friends they've all known each other as I have, almost since we were kids, you know? So the relationship among my group of friends [there] is a healthy relationship"* (Ibidem). Moreover, in this case, neither is it a complicity created around consumption: *"My group of friends [there] includes people who have been into it and aren't any more, people who still are [and] only use once in a while, and people who have never been into it."* (Ibidem) The "healthy relationship" translates into a relationship of respect (for each other's choices) and trust.

However, if friendship can constitute a criterion for confidentiality [*"Out of my friends, everybody knows. No, I don't hide it"* (E3/R98)], it may not be enough: *"So, it's only my friends who know, and not everybody, some of them... it's like this: my colleagues here at the Faculty, these friends of mine no, they've never, never known... in my work environment obviously not! The ones who knew were my friends from where I'm from and in [the neighbourhood] ..."* (E1/R63). The reason for excluding certain friends from knowledge is that they *"aren't within the context"* (Ibidem); *"only... with people who know what the experience is like, right?"* (E7/R143).

But insofar as the secrecy varies according to whether or not the other is within the "context", this can mean that a distinction is made within the group of confidants depending on the substance: *"Here [in the city], when I smoke hashish, I'm really at ease... With LSD it's only with friends, only with experienced people, not with non-drug users, because they have no idea and can't know about it."* (E19/R160, 260) In general, they also can't know about the *"other heavy drugs, because they're passing situations..."* (Ibidem).

The latter argument also enters into a strategy of hiding the behaviour from oneself: *"As I'm at a stage where this doesn't go any further, as I spend per week [range of amounts], so I won't worry any more about this..."* (E23/R91); *"But also, okay, we're talking about using, but I don't use drugs anyway, I don't turn drugs into daily use or anything. I take it as a bit of a joke, don't I?"* (E3/R38).

Family relationships

If care is taken in the delimitation of confidentiality among friends, in the family context or around the family the mobilisation of dissimulation strategies requires an even more intense investment. This investment must, however, be weighed up taking into account the consumption cultures and scenarios. For example, family intimacy, which may extend beyond the domestic space, decisively marks the use of cannabinoids integrated into family routines. The domestic space can also be a refuge for heroin users at different stages of their consumption but, at least when we consider it in terms of its traditional functions, it is not much associated with consumption aimed at social contact or relationships.

Besides the way in which the family space can be associated with particular consumption cultures or scenarios, the family now interests us more particularly as a social space regulating the different normative orders. In this sense, the importance of the family as an object of strategies of dissimulation derives from its central role of socialisation and management of expectations and social identities. To give a full account of this importance, we shall first of all analyse situations in which secrecy does not exist, that is to say situations in which, in some way, attempts to hide behaviour not conforming to the expectations of others, in the light of the referential of normative conformity, have been frustrated. We are then interested in outlining the social space of confidentiality within the family. In particular, we want to know whether secrecy is associated with certain types of bonds and what motivates these preferences.

Absence of secrecy or the limits of dissimulation

In order to gather evidence to answer these questions, we shall start by analysing situations in which there is no secrecy, hoping that, by contrast, they will allow us to better understand the situations shaped by strategies of dissimulation. The biographies collected reveal four types of situations: 1) rupture, as a definitive milestone in a process of disaffiliation; 2) support, as a testimony of solidarity; 3) protection, as a reinforcement of the socialising role of the family; and 4) stopping consumption, so as not to cause moral damage. These four situations point to family contexts with very different socialising orientations, but what we are particularly interested in underscoring is the fact that a strategy of dissimulation means, in the first place, in relation to the intentionalities of the individuals. These intentionalities are motivated by values that are important for individuals but at which the objective circumstances of the situations often do not let us guess. As we have seen above, strategies of secrecy are always equivocal (hiding is partial, from some people, in certain circumstances...) to the extent of the ambivalence of the gazes that are crossed and of the diffractive density of the situations. These strategies therefore take on different meanings when we consider them in relation to the consumption cultures and scenarios or to the positions taken in relation to the normative frameworks in force.

The first situation occurs when secrecy is no longer possible, because "the emperor has no clothes" and there is nothing left to hide. In this type of biography, consumption behaviours go wrong, leading to a progressive break with conventional social ties and, in many cases, even a break with the social ties that replaced them in the course of consumption trajectories. As Robert Castel would say, it is a process of disaffiliation from traditional protective ties. This means that ruptures are not consummated all at once and that strategies enabling consumption are not defined from the outset but are forged through the particularities of the pathways. This is also why strategies of concealment are dynamic in time, flexible according to the circumstances and differentiated according to the people from whom one is hiding. And this happens both from the consumer's perspective and from the perspective of his relationships, namely his relatives. A quick sketch of a process of disaffiliation, from the consumer's perspective, allows us to pinpoint some significant moments.

In another work[26], produced from the same materials, we were able to see that the meaning attributed by individuals to the first consumption is not that of transgression of the rules, but rather of curiosity, the spirit of adventure, a game... Contrary to what happens in the vast majority of cases, in the population we interviewed the first consumption was followed by more! A first consumption can be hidden, because at the very least it is considered an act of rebellion... but it can be communicated, especially to parents. In some cases, what is hidden is not the first consumption (generally of hashish) but those that follow.

From the moment that people learn to like consuming, as H. Becker (1985) puts it, it is possible that, initially, individuals hide their consumption from themselves. The end of secrecy begins when one acknowledges to oneself that the consumption is not just a "bit of fun" [*"But I don't use drugs anyway, I don't turn drugs into daily use or anything. I take it as a bit of fun, don't I?"* (E3/R38)], that it has consequences [*"I'm outside that world, in a way, right, because when I do use, that world doesn't affect me at all, you know?"* (E6/R30)] and that a hierarchy of risks can be constructed [*"It's like cigarettes, I also know that it can cause cancer in me and that it's bad for my health, but I continue to smoke aware of that"* (E1/R61); *"Alcohol,*

---

[26] *Construção de espaços de transgressão: o consumo de drogas* (Ibidem).

caffeine, tobacco itself, that's all drugs, everything is bad for me, you know?" (E6/R45)].

One of the consumption biographies that we collected marks out the path that can be travelled in this type of trajectory:

> *"At the beginning when I started using [heroin; before that, other drugs were already used] I think I did it to have fun... it was at the weekend, it was like that, once in a while, once a month at the most. Sometimes quite a long time went by without even... thinking about it... It was all a very gradual evolution. Things went on and on and on. When it got a bit faster, when it became a constant thing, there was always an excuse to do it... And it became a reality, I needed to consume... it became a necessity... I lost interest in everything... You don't think about anything, there's no reasoning... People would call me to arrange things... and I would make up lame excuses that at first still stuck, because nobody knew, but then they started not sticking and people started confronting me and I had to tell them the truth."* (E1/R38-42)

The idiosyncrasies of individual trajectories result in a multiplicity of scenarios of the phase that follows and from which one can no longer hide things. From the perspective of close family, perhaps this corresponds to a phase that can no longer be ignored. In cases of rupture with the family setting, which is frequent, and without institutional support (less probable in more recent times) disaffiliation is consummated and the accounts expose, in the raw, the wounds associated with behaviour that cannot be hidden (cf. dependence scenario above).

In a second variant of situations of dependence, disaffiliation is not completely realised because the family setting continues to be a support, either intermittently [*"Many cures were imposed by my mother ... others were because I was living on the street and was sick of being hungry, of being cold, of living in those conditions and I would take the initiative and go home"* (E16/R87)], or because the consumption can take place at home [*"[Name of husband] was a heroin user for five years, here at home ... And the family, which was that lady heroin, because that's a real family ... With heroin addicts the only thing that's always there for them is heroin, they have nothing else"* (E8/R81)].

A third situation that seems significant to us in terms of the importance that the family setting can have in consumption trajectories is reported by

Interviewee 1 who, having reached a stage in her consumption journey where she has to "tell the truth" (see above), decides to stop using (heroin at least) in order not to have to cause her parents grief in this way: *"Although I had never really told my parents I was using, I stopped using on my own initiative so they would never know"* (E1/R59). This expression of compassion can thus unfold the feelings of respect or submission associated with parental authority.

The socialising and protective function usually attributed to the family setting can also be observed in situations in which the abstinence norm is not followed or at least not followed indiscriminately. In one of the cases we observed, after consumption of other substances is stopped, the use of cannabis is integrated into daily or occasional family rituals and upheld as a way of life (cf. above). The socialisation of the child into this type of consumption and its integration in the family setting are justified by the protection they can bring: *"We had to take that option because [Name] grew up seeing a kid like him... selling joints... We were in doubt whether to talk to him about our way of life, or whether we would not mention it and say it was no good or something, try to inhibit him... But he said that he smoked, and after a while, we decided: 'It's better for you to smoke with us than to smoke outside' and it was on that condition that our cohesion developed"* (E4/R14-15). Thus, neither the family as an institution nor family settings can be considered homogeneous where abstinence is concerned, thus revealing a margin of strategy on the part of drug users.

The challenges posed by drug use are good analysers for the knowledge of family relationships, particularly their orientations towards values and the ways these are managed within intra-family relationships. The fears associated with drug use and the dramatic representation of its consequences strain relationships and force a tense mobilisation of moral dimensions.

This mobilisation involves all the parties in the relationships, although in different ways, according to the positions (of authority, proximity...) assumed. The consequences may also be more or less serious for the partners, ranging from support to exclusion. Preferring to have a dead son to a son addicted to drugs ["[My father] said that to have a son who was a drug addict he wanted to have a dead son first, at least he would have the pain only once" (E15/R230)] does not assume less serious proportions than the radical exclusion of the drug user from the family ["When everything started to fall apart I ask for help, I thought that by going back to my parents' house I would manage, and probably I even did, if I went back to those principles, to that environment I was used to before, I could pull the cassette back and then I would take the course and stuff, but they rejected it" (E23/R36)] or the lasting exclusion ["They cut it off. Today they don't talk to me" (Ibidem)] and definitive ["I never thought they would get angry with me definitely" (E23/R11-12]).

Hiding from whom

The constraints associated with consumption and its consequences can give us a measure of the reasons why drug users may hide within the family setting.

On the one hand, consumption is considered to betray the bonds of trust and an image of conformity constructed in the family setting: *"Who wouldn't I want to know? My parents, first of all, obviously, but it's not for fear that they would throw me out of the house or that the relationship would be bad, it was because that knowledge, you know, would be such a disappointment for them..."* (E6/R124); *"People end up forming another opinion right from that moment [when they become aware]. They look at the person, well, that girl takes drugs, she's no longer the person we thought she was."* (E36/R93). The importance attributed to consumption in evaluating all other dimensions of a person's life is rejected by drug users: *"Because I did that, I was going to be such a disappointment to them, but as it never changed my life it was going to be a disappointment based on almost nothing, you know?* (E6/R124); *"It's not that I hide because I think I shouldn't present myself like that in front of people or that people will think I'm this or that or the other. No, it's because my use doesn't justify it, it's not even an element in my life that has a meaning beyond what it is, which is circumstantial" (E31/R53); "There are some cases where it's maybe better not to say anything... If I now [say] 'Grandma, I smoke a few joints and whatever...', well, she'd think that I was completely ruined (laughs)"* (E12/R100).

On the other hand, dissimulation can also be justified by affective reasons: *"[My grandmother] is already old, if she knew I think she would be very sad."* (E12/R100); *"No [I say]. Hey, man, why am I going to give my mother a headache?"* (E33/R121).

It is clear that knowledge of consumption not only intervenes on the levels of identities or on the affective level, since it may also compromise the relationship and condition the family's way of life, including, as we saw above, access to family resources: *"I try not to make too much effort, but sometimes it is a bit bad, it is a bit ugly... also out of disrespect, it shocks people, you have to take that into account... But it is not because they know me or not, it is precisely because it can shock their own sensibility, that's all. Consequently, it was going to shock me, because they were going to bother me..."* (E32/R66).

The fear of a rupture or a deterioration of the affective relationship, as a result of distrust and the controls that the knowledge of consumption could represent, may also justify hiding it: *"On the one hand, I would actually like my parents to know, because I've always talked to them about everything. It was, well, for them to have an idea, but, all the same, I also wouldn't like it because then comes that constant pressure that always ends up being behind you."* (E1/R65). This desire to create channels of communication may lead to a strategy of "testing the waters": *"I always tried to talk about it, you know, never saying that I was doing it, but trying to talk about these issues to see if one day I could say that I consume, you know? Like testing the waters."* (E10/R46).

Between the social and affective reasons for dissimulation there is a normative barrier that is considered to be difficult to overcome. This gulf can be attributed to a lack of "literacy" [*"There was never a big investment in literacy, people are still very... lots of people are dumb! It's not a question of being dumb, no... hey, man, they don't read newspapers, they don't watch debates, many don't know how to read and write, you know?"* (E6/R61)] or to a lack of knowledge of consumption cultures: *"My mother never knew... We'd roll a joint around her and she might not even know what we're doing. So, her register... She has no idea of this kind of knowledge"* (E4/R15).

The interviewees consider that this distance limits the possibilities of communication: *"Let's say that I, with my parents, in that aspect... there's a break there [...]. From there on they don't know anything more about my life, because they don't understand..."* (E36/R91); *"I think they're people who would never understand and would never accept it, so it's not even worth getting into arguments about it because it's really not worth it!"* (E10/R151); *"I'm never going to be able to say it, nor am I going to be able to make them understand what I feel and the good motivations that I might possibly have for my use..."* (E32/R122). This limitation can be elevated to a dramatic register: *"There are those for whom the perspective of drugs is so drastic that it is not worth telling them that you smoke."* (E4/R36).

Concealment can be aimed at any family member, including the extended family, for the reasons described above and according to very variable circumstances or considerations of convenience. The only relationship that seems to us to be better preserved is the one that drug users have with their parents and, after that, with their grandparents. Parents and grandparents are, indeed, with rare exceptions, systematically cited as not being allowed to know about consumption: *"No, the people who really can't know, who I really don't want to know, are my parents, obviously"* (E2/R110, E17); *"They don't know, nor do I want them to know, no, you see? Nor do I want them to know, of course"* (E6/R30); *"My parents, of course not! They couldn't know and it wouldn't be good for them to know, nor does it make sense for them to know!... My parents and all the rest of my family"* (E31/R51).

This secrecy in relation to parents may, in fact, remain even when the relationship is open and characterised by trust: *"My father is somewhat interested in this and we talk about it with a certain ease, but I always don't mention the idea that I'm still using hashish, or anything else..."* (E4/R9); *"My grandfather, I don't know... he's really weird. There was never any conversation, he talks and talks and talks. I don't know, but I can't say for sure. As a matter of respect, I never told him"* (E15/R244).

We know that, in addition to affective or moral considerations, dissimulation may also be motivated by defence of drug users' self-interest, their individual comfort or their reasons for using drugs: *"The question of 'who couldn't know' is very subjective, you know? Because it's like this: if I knew that [if] my parents found out that I had ever done that they would throw me out, then my parents couldn't know"* (E6/R124).

Spaces where hiding takes place

To be able to think about the spaces or places where consumption is hidden, we must first of all place ourselves in the perspective of the normative orders that promote abstinence and which are therefore silent about the spaces where consumption occurs (not considering the health strategies of assisted consumption within the scope of harm reduction strategies, which fall outside the scope of our purpose). This means that, in order to understand which the spaces are that are chosen for hiding, we have to consider the very strategies put into practice by drug users, who in principle are faced with the situation of not being able to consume anywhere. Under these conditions, the solutions we have identified seem to us to be linked to two different but interconnected types of legitimacy: on the one hand, secrecy practices are regulated by consumer cultures; on the other, they owe much to circumstances regulated by the intentionality of individuals themselves.

Spaces associated with consumption scenarios and cultures

The data that we have available from other sources[27] show us that circumstances exist in which certain types of consumption are more frequent: rituals of initiation or of transition and festive or recreational moments, for example. From this point of view, each substance appears associated with a certain "set of specifications"[28] (or responds to a specific injunction to consume), has its own modus operandi and produces specific effects that only the initiated are considered to be capable of sharing. Certain types of space may appear to be associated in a privileged way with these requirements: for example, when consumption is linked to "curiosity" or "rebellion" the spaces invested have some symbolism of transgression ("behind the houses", in abandoned or secluded spaces...). For some, recreational consumption takes place in places which seem obvious: *"For a while I dedicated myself to the use of ecstasy and LSD, going to so-called raves, by association, obviously"* (E1/R33). However, a rave does not delimit its own space, because it is not a space, but a place that is collectively constructed by the meanings that the actors lend it to assume a specific valence: *"Usually we try to go to places, I don't know, that have nothing to do with this, right? In terms more..., in terms of nature... where you can be at ease, beaches... places where you are more at peace, where there is less*

---

[27] Cf. in particular the results of our studies of the general population through the INPG.

[28] Expression that we use in preference to "motivations", taking our lead from one of our interviewees who queried the formulation of a question around "motivations for consumption" as proof of our ignorance about the world of consumption which, according to him, was not regulated by our rationality.

chance of there being some kind of bother." (E7/R107) Other types of consumption that are less dependent on facilitating scenarios may take place in spaces of exclusion where, just like other "deviant" practices, they are more tolerated by the instances of control[29].

However, none of these consumption spaces has, in itself, any relation with secrecy: they are only associated with consumption when they are symbolically invested for it, and many other uses are possible in them; on the other hand, their potential for dissimulation is very relative, and in certain circumstances where there is concealment one could say that "the cat is out of the bag".

The loose relation between consumption and space can be further questioned based on the "consumption scenarios" that we analysed above. From this point of view, there may be an elective relation between each scenario and privileged spaces, depending for example on whether the locus of consumption is more public or private. However, once again, none of the spaces or places likely to be associated with a scenario itself hides or lets us see independent of the intentionality of the consumer.

This means that in order to understand concealment we must take into account the consumption cultures or scenarios, which are leveraged by the drug users' intentionality. This intentionality can only be understood when we consider the construction of social relations of dissimulation, as we sought to show above.

Space as instrument of intentionality

Thus, if consumption scenarios, because of the cultures they represent in relation to substances, explain why certain spaces are more likely to be used for consumption than others, it is also the case, as we have shown in another work[30], that even in this circumstance, the dimensions that delimit these cultures can be constructed, as happens for example with the categories of

---

[29] Cf. our work on spaces of exclusion: Balsa, Casimiro, "A exclusão e o espaço, espaços de exclusão", in Casimiro Balsa (Ed.), *Relações sociais de espaço — Homenagem a Jean Remy*, Col. CEOS/Inquéritos – 4, Edições Colibri/CEOS, Lisbon, 2006, pp. 13-33.

[30] Balsa, Casimiro. "A construção de espaços de transgressão: o consumo de drogas", in António Dimas Cardoso e Domingos Vaz (Orgs.), *Cidades, Escalas e Transações*, Col. Navegar é Preciso. Vila Nova de Famalicão: Húmus, 2021, pp. 40-87.

"public" or "private" space. This means that certain physical and "objective" spaces may be given quite different meanings. This constructed character of consumption spaces is even more evident when we consider spaces of first consumption. More evident is the construction of a geography of representations of the self, which allow us to distinguish "being oneself", when one is not using, from being "outside oneself", when using, or even to distinguish between "being up" and "being down" in relation to states associated with consumption (Balsa, 2022). The definition of spaces of dissimulation depends thus on the very circumstances in which this takes place, with it understood that the valence of a certain space may change according to the people who inhabit it. We also saw above, in considering the semantics of secrecy itself, that the need to mobilise the space may be more or less important according to what one wants to hide, the act of consumption itself, its signs and its consequences.

The observation that seems most significant to us, however, has to do with the fact that in some orientations of the choices reported to us, space is never a determining factor in defining strategies of concealment. In fact, it seems to us that there is no single determining factor when one wants to hide consumption. Rather, there is a decision situation in which there is an intentionality (to hide), in a particular circumstance of consumption and consumption trajectory, and strategies, modalities and the very means to hide. The space is one of these modalities but is only relevant when combined with the other elements that participate in the decision to dissimulate.

In other words, from the perspective of concealing consumption, any space may be selected: *"I think alcohol and pot, it can be anywhere and even with people who don't even smoke and don't drink"* (E27/R53); *"Then we go anywhere. But I don't make a big distinction because... drugs are consumed anywhere"* (E35/R17); *"Depending on what you feel like, you can get it easily anywhere"* (E37/R48). However, the choice of place is not made randomly, but taking into consideration all the elements that intervene in the decision situation. Thus, it seems "obvious" to someone that smoking a joint or injecting heroin are not done in the same spaces: *"Obviously, having a joint can be done just like that outdoors, sometimes sitting on park benches... while using heroin it's not here [work city] that I do it, and when I do it's in the privacy of my home or someone else's home, or if there are no homes... cars or another hidden place."* (E1/R14). The spaces where hashish is smoked are different if the consumption takes place in a perspective of discovery or transgression, or if it is part of a life routine or a ritual of sociability. In some cases, the domestic space is the appropriate place, in others, the rule is *"no smoking joints at home"* (E32/R66).

The relationship of consumption with the space is not, however, limited to consumption as such; dissimulation may extend to all moments involving consumption (acquisition, the frequenting of places, or socialising with people associated with consumption...) and to its effects. This extension requires that the practices of dissimulation, especially when the goal is to "eliminate the signs", multiply in different spaces, according to what one wants to hide and from whom, confirming the idea that it is people and the social relations established that are decisive in establishing the meanings that the space takes on in strategies of dissimulation.

Conclusion: ethics as index, in the final instance, of social relations of dissimulation

In a first approximation, we have to admit that the normative referential instituted on consumption imposes that the secret be kept (see above). Indeed, let us take one thing for granted in our observation: people hide something, for the simple reason that they cannot show it and, when they do show it, it is above all when they have nothing else to lose. What is at issue here, then, is not so much whether they hide as the reasons why they do so. But given that they have to hide, for reasons of legal compliance and social convenience, other questions arise that are of interest to us, namely: on the one hand, what modalities of dissimulation are adopted and, on the other, under what circumstances these strategies may vary and what social meanings this variation may have.

In this section we have tried to answer these questions by identifying the elements through which the strategies of dissimulation take shape, having considered essentially the contexts or the people, the modalities and the circumstances of time and space. These circumstances do not occur only at the moment of intention to hide consumption, but also extend to preliminary activities (acquisition, coexistence with specific groups or the frequenting of certain spaces...) and to the effects of consumption (for example, in the family or professional setting).

The interpretative hypothesis that we want to propose has to do precisely with these elements. In a first approximation, it seems reasonable to think that it would be possible to outline a social cartography of secrecy that would make plain the contexts or people from whom one hides (or not) and the circumstances of time and space in which this is done. While being unable to aim here at probabilistic knowledge, the idea would be to identify the most significant associations that might allow us to conceptualise an architecture of secrecy. However, while we were able to construct some ideal types of the relations of dissimulation, it was not easy to establish an unambiguous pattern when considered from the point of view of individual strategies. We believe that the problem is not in the materials, but in the complexity and unpredictability of the strategies of dissimulation.

Indeed, the general idea that we draw from the analysis of these materials is that practices of dissimulation are not linked, in principle, to any of the modalities of the dimensions—space, people or circumstances—that arc able to substantiate them. Thus, none of these modalities appears to be particularly strongly associated with any strategy of dissimulation. In other words, practices of secrecy may mobilise any type of space, be exercised in any circumstance or target any person. This means that it is not possible to predict strategies of concealment based only on knowledge of the dimensions that consubstantiate them. We believe that this predictability—and thus the meaning of the modalities of concealment and of the above-mentioned architecture of secrecy—may reside in the intentionality of individuals, regulated by the nature of affective relations and by the management of the effects that knowledge of consumption could have on those from whom it is hidden. As already mentioned, this framework embodies well the intuition with which Fredrik Barth circumvented the functionalist postulate (cf. "Preface 1998", Barth 1998), suggesting that it is the intentionality of the actors that gives meaning to the markers of their positions, and not the other way around.

When it comes to understanding the unpredictability of relations of dissimulation, it seems to us that strategies are first of all linked to an ethics of relations (that is to say, to ethical orientations of "ways of life"), before attaching themselves to the supports of the relationship (from whom one hides, where one hides, under what circumstances one hides). These supports intervene in secrecy practices in a relatively random way, that is they seem to have some plasticity when we consider the effects they may exert. For this very reason, the exception that we find to this unpredictability—the recurring concern with the dissimulation of consumption, first of all with regard to parents and secondly with regard to grandparents—confirms the importance that the ethics of relations may have in regulating relations of dissimulation.

We therefore formulate the hypothesis that an understanding of the strategies of concealment requires a model that enables us to integrate 1) on the one hand, the criteria that guide the decisions that individuals take when faced with normative reference frameworks and consumption scenarios and 2) on the other hand, the decision to hide or to show, which has above all to do with the ethics of social relations that individuals adopt in their conduct of life[31]. What seems to us to be at stake on this last level is the way in which the socio-affective resources of relationships are mobilised. Moreover, dissimulation allows these resources to be regulated in such a way that they can produce effects in both directions in a relationship, although these directions are not necessarily the same: 1) dissimulating so as not to hurt the positions or sensibilities of significant others and 2) dissimulating so as not to call into question a position or a self-identity that one wishes to value.

[31] The distinction between "dispositions" (in conjunction with structures) and "life conducts" (through which individuals impose themselves as agents) was placed by Max Weber at the basis of his project for a comprehensive sociology, according to the analysis proposed by Catherine Calliot-Thélène (Colliot-Thélène 2006).

CHAPTER 3

MEDIATION BETWEEN OBSERVABLE AND OBSERVED VALIDATION OF RESULTS AND RECONFIGURATION OF "GENERAL POPULATION"[32]

Presentation

The results of the third General Population Survey, applied in 2012, are excellent from the perspective of an assessment of the public policies that have been developed in Portugal under the banner of decriminalisation, with integrated action in the field of diagnosis, prevention, supply reduction, demand reduction, harm reduction, treatment and reintegration of populations likely to be affected or who are already affected by the use of drugs, both licit and illicit. In fact, after a slight increase, from 7.8% to 12%, between the first two application periods of the Survey—2001 and 2007—the lifetime prevalence of any illicit drug had by 2012 dropped to 9.5%. This decrease can be seen, with few exceptions, in all substances—licit and illicit—and is also observed in the other time periods used to measure prevalence: use in the last year and in the last month. The variations observed also follow, more or less, the same pattern: rates of prevalence in 2012 are between those observed in 2001 and 2007, that is higher than the former and lower than the latter. The main propensities in consumption, as clarified in previous studies, remain when we consider consequences or situations of dependence, and it is also worth noting that the closer

[32] Based on the chapter on "discussion of the results" of the third application of the National survey on drug use among general population, conducted in 2012 (Balsa, C., C. Vital and C. Urbano. 2014. *Inquérito Nacional ao Consumo de Substâncias Psicoativas na População Geral, Portugal 2012*. Lisbon: SICAD — Serviço de Intervenção nos Comportamentos Aditivos e nas Dependências).

relationship already observed between male and female behaviour has become stronger.

Adopting a position of prudence, motivated by the principle of realism summarised in the margins of error[33], these reductions in prevalence rates could be read, at the very least, as a stabilisation of consumption. The problem, however, is not so much in the degree to which this more or less optimistic this interpretation is well founded. The problem lies in the fact that rates of prevalence could not have stabilised, let alone fallen.

When we presented the results of the application of the study in 2007, we justified the extent of the increase observed then by considering, in addition to the maintenance of consumption cultures (Balsa et al. 2008), a cohort effect, according to which prevalence can rise regardless of consumption behaviour. However, taking into account the history of consumption in Portugal, the cohort effect should lead to an increase in lifetime prevalence, even assuming that consumption had remained stable.

The unexpected result we obtained leads us to detail and share the discussion of an operation that always concerns us within our production space that is motivated by the question of knowing "how could we be wrong" when we present a given result. To this end, we shall undertake our interrogations through the following steps:

- First, we shall question the cohort effect itself and the conditions under which it can occur;
- then, we shall report on the operations that allowed us to (in)validate our methodology and the information collection procedures (validity);
- also, on a methodological level, we shall question the capacity of our measuring instrument to collect reliable information over successive applications (reliability);
- finally, following on from Chapter 1, we shall question the category of "general population" itself.

---

[33] Due to financial constraints, the sample size for the 2012 application was about half of what is usual for the study—15,000 individuals in 2001 and 12,000 in 2007, 2016 and 2021—increasing the margins of error.

The cohort effect

Considering the possibility of measuring the lifetime prevalence of a given population's behaviour regarding the use of psychoactive substances, the cohort effect is explained by the fact that substance use by a person or population at a given time is recorded in their life biography in such a way that, in a later period and until they leave that population, it allows them to be classified in the group of "lifetime users". It is for this reason that the prevalence of lifetime consumption is presented as a stock or cumulative variable: it tots up declarations of consumption over the years, just so long as individuals do not forget to declare them at a given time...

Let us take the example of a study on the lifetime prevalence of use of psychoactive substance, carried out in 2007 on the whole Portuguese population of people born between 1943 and 1992, so aged between 15 and 64 at the time of the study. After obtaining the results, we know that the average prevalence is 11.9%. It is to be expected that, since drug use is a cultural phenomenon, each of the age cohorts covered by the study contributes with a different weight to this average score. Thus, we observe that the oldest cohort, the one with people aged between 60 and 64, has a very small weight (0.7%). By contrast, the youngest cohorts contribute to the result with greater weight (21.2% for the group of those aged 20 to 24), and intermediate groups with a decreasing weight as age increases.

What is expected to happen, when the study is repeated five years later, maintaining the same limits of the reference population (15-64 years)? Now the lower and upper bounds of the birth years of the target population move to 1948 (people aged 64) and 1997 (people aged 15) respectively. This means that the people who made up the cohort with very low consumption prevalence have left the population, and a new cohort of young people has entered that, if consumption is maintained at the level observed in the previous survey, has much higher prevalence rates. This substitution of cohorts with different consumption behaviours means that average prevalence rates tend to increase according to the weight in the total population of the respective cohorts. Thus, as older populations leave the study population, the average prevalence rate increases, approaching the rates observed in the age cohorts of those who consume more. This progressive increase in prevalence is expected until the older populations, that is those who have not participated in cultures conducive to consumption, have left the study population.

What are the conditions for this cohort effect not to occur, that is, for there not to be a trend for a progressive increase in prevalence rates "throughout life"? In the first instance, we shall limit ourselves to the variables that constitute the cohort effect itself.

1. So long as cultural and normative models related to consumption behaviours do not change substantially, the cohort effect will only occur while a gap remains in terms of experiences between the different age groups considered in a given reference universe. Thus, in countries where consumption cultures, even if of different substances, are longer established, to the point where older groups have had the same opportunities to consume as today's young people, the cohort effect will not occur. We believe this to be the case in countries such as France, the United Kingdom or Germany. It is certainly not the case in Portugal. The first Survey of the General Population, carried out in 2001, shows that declarations of the use of any substance begin to be substantial (7.7%) from the cohort born between 1957 and 1966 (aged between 35 and 44), that is individuals who were aged 15 between 1972 and 1981. In the oldest cohort (aged 45 to 54), comprising those born between 1947 and 1956, and so aged 15 between 1962 and 1971, declarations of consumption drop to 2.2%, and in the oldest age group (55 to 64) only 0.4% of the population declare any consumption. We can thus affirm that the use of any illicit substance starts to become more frequent from the 1970s onwards, probably as changes in the political regime opened up the possibility of cultural practices or manifestations associated with the use of illicit substances. Returning to the 35 to 44 age group in the 2001 application, where we believe is the cut-off line between more and less frequent use, we see that in the subgroup of individuals who were aged 15 in the period 1977-1981, the youngest—those who turned 15 after 1976 (the 35-39 age group)—present prevalence rates clearly higher than those of the next group, the bulk of whose adolescence was before Portugal's 1974 Revolution (and who turned 19 in 1976): 10.6% against 4.6%. Considering that the 35-39 age

group is in fact the cut-off line, we can see in the following table that, in an application of the study carried out in 2013 they would have constituted the 50-54 age group, but only in an application carried out in 2023 would they top the range of the reference universe (at 60-65), so that only from then on would their substitution by a group at the bottom of the range (aged 15-19) no longer produce a cohort effect, or it would produce only a moderate effect, depending on the greater or lesser proximity of the rates of prevalence recorded between the two groups (and the two periods) considered.

2. Based on the results obtained in 2007, we can estimate the increase that would be caused in the average prevalence, measured in 2012, by simply replacing the group of 60- to 64-year-olds by the group of 15- to 19-year-olds in 2012, taking the consumption rates of the latter at the level observed in 2007. Under these conditions, that is, without considering the influence of any additional variables, the cohort effect would have raised the average prevalence of lifetime consumption in 2012 from 11.9% to 12.6%.

3. It should also be noted that the cut-off group is preceded by older groups that, especially in the case of those closer together, may have lower but not negligible rates of prevalence. This means that, as the individuals with more significant rates of prevalence get older, the cohort effect gets smaller. It should also be noted that in our example we considered the consumption rates of the youngest group (aged 15-19), but this is not the group that records the highest rates of prevalence. These are recorded for the 20-24 age group — with a rate of around 21% in 2007, which would point to the average prevalence level for the general population to be reached when the cohort effect has exhausted its effects, if there has been no significant change in patterns of use in the meantime.

4. The cohort effect therefore assumes that there is a significant difference in terms of consumption in the new groups entering the reference population (in our case, individuals aged between 15 and 19), in relation to that of the older groups leaving this population (for

example, aged 60-65), which tend to have lower consumption. If this condition does not occur, or from the moment it does not occur, average prevalence rates in the universe may not increase, increase more moderately or even start to decrease. In the case of prevalence in Portugal, through the three successive applications of the study—2001, 2007 and 2012—we see that prevalence rates in the youngest group (aged 15-19) record successive falls, from 10.9% through 8.6% to 7.5%. In the last application, moreover, prevalence rates are down for all individuals in the "young adults" group (15- to 34-year-olds). This means that, with these trends, the size of the cohort effect will tend to diminish but never disappear, since the older age groups that have been replaced by these newcomers have very low prevalence rates.

5. Of course, the cohort effect can be altered if we modify the age limits of the reference population. Indeed, if we for example change the boundaries of the study population to extend it to people aged 65-74, this will extend the time needed for prevalence to homogenise on the basis of higher rates. To the extent that these groups have still lower or even zero prevalence rates, this will also lead to a reduction in average prevalence rates.

Table 3-1. Evolution of age cohorts, through different possible survey years

Years of birth	Years in which aged 15-19	Ages in 2001	Ages in 2005	Ages in 2009	Ages in 2013	Ages in 2017	Ages in 2021
1937-1941	1952-1956	60-64	65-69	70-74	75-79	80-84	85-89
1942-1946	1957-1961	55-59	60-64	65-69	70-74	75-79	80-84
1947-1951	1962-1966	50-54	55-59	60-64	65-69	70-74	75-79
1952-1956	1967-1971	45-49	50-54	55-59	60-64	65-69	70-74
1957-1961	1972-1976	40-44	45-49	50-54	55-59	60-64	65-69
1962-1966	1977-1981	35-39	40-44	45-49	50-54	55-59	60-64
1967-1971	1982-1986	30-34	35-39	40-44	45-49	50-54	55-59
1972-1976	1987-1991	25-29	30-34	35-39	40-44	45-49	50-54
1977-1981	1992-1996	20-24	25-29	30-34	35-39	40-44	45-49
1982-1986	1997-2001	15-19	20-24	25-29	30-34	35-39	40-44
1987-1991	2002-2006	--	15-19	20-24	25-29	30-34	35-39
1992-1996	2007-2011	--	--	15-19	20-24	25-29	30-34
1997-2001	2012-2016	--	--	--	15-19	20-24	25-29
2002-2006	--	--	--	--	--	15-19	20-24
2007-2011	--	--	--	--	--	--	15-19

Methodology and information gathering procedures: validity

The reduction in prevalence that we are discussing here must also be analysed from the point of view of technical and methodological issues, since this is the level of production of results for which the team of researchers has the greatest responsibility. The first question we may ask ourselves here has to do with the validity of our questionnaire, that is to say, to determine how suitable our instrument of observation is for measuring the behaviour that it aims to apprehend. More than a rhetorical or ritual question about the role of those who undertake extensive data collection, this is one that should always be present in the concerns of the researcher, since we believe that the instruments of measurement, as the constructions that they are (and constructions oriented according to different representations of the problems studied) have only a certain probability of approximating the situations that are themselves very much coloured by the circumstances in which they occur. Following what we said in previous chapters, we fully acknowledge all the constraints that may aggravate this distance between the universe of the survey and the universe of respondents — constraints that arise from the fact that we are working with a measuring instrument that is closed (and therefore not very sensitive in capturing singularities) and quite standardised in line with the methodology of international comparative research (and so more focused on the transnational expression of situations than on their local manifestations). The questions of validity that we wish to raise go beyond these constraints, which we have already discussed. In addition to dealing with the individual idiosyncrasies with which we are used to coping, it is a matter of knowing to what extent responses to a survey that aims to study hidden behaviours may be altered, over time, according to changes in normative orientations that may change the way these behaviours are evaluated. In particular, we may ask whether the crisis that Portugal has gone through since the end of the previous study (2007) might have changed the models of justification, if not the very order of values that may frame the social judgment of a behaviour that, while decriminalised, is not therefore any less socially and legally proscribed.

1. In order for this change in the models of justification to help clear up our problem, we must hypothesise that normative orientations in times of crisis—which bring generalised restrictions and appeal to feelings of restraint and prudence, or even guilt—would lead people who had previously declared some consumption to "forget" that they consumed, that is, they would prefer not to confront a situation of cognitive dissonance, even if this dissonance related to different moments in their experience. This "forgetfulness" could thus justify the reduction in prevalence that we have been discussing.

2. In favour of this hypothesis we can draw on the results presented in previous chapters that have shown us, in essence, that the positions regarding the confidentiality of consumption vary according to the substances themselves, to the assessment made of the regulatory framework, to the assessment of one's own relationship with consumption, to the relationship of proximity/distance with people that might be informed, to the proximity/distance of these people to/from consumption cultures, or to the circumstances (space/time) in which the information is provided. Making it more difficult to determine the conditions of confidentiality is the fact that the co-

occurrence of some of these factors does not lead to convergent communication decisions (for example, friends may or may not be informed, depending on whether or not they are considered to have a "culture" of consumption...). Thus, in addition to being associated with privileged spaces, places and times (as shown in our studies), consumption is also marked by normative contexts on the basis of which confidentiality networks are designed that define the potential of listening attributed to the people who are part of them, designing spaces of complicity, through which drug users move, and spaces of guilt, from which they keep away.

3. Can the decision to report a consumption behaviour be considered less compromising when the "confidant" is an employee of a polling company? We do not have the information to answer this question. What we do know is that the construction of the conditions of observation tends to invest this employee with a status that allows him/her to listen in a neutral way, that is, neither complicit nor accusing. This listening is also defined as non-committal for the informant (cf. technical modalities of survey questioning). In our case, the interviewer is also previously invested, through a letter of introduction, with an institutional legitimacy (the University) and a mission justified by a social purpose.

4. Thus, we have two apparently contradictory orders of arguments regarding the validity of our measuring instrument.
    a) On the one hand, the communication of consumption is subject to confidentiality strategies marked by normative contexts. However, in order for us to assume that the reduction in prevalence that we recorded is due to the control of respondents over their answers, according to a change in the normative context, we would have to know if this change of context actually exists and, if so, if the population had internalised it in their representation models and materialised it in their responses, and to what extent. Our study does not allow us to clarify these orientations.

b) On the other hand, the ambition of the scientific community is to build observation conditions capable of ensuring total transparency between consumption and the respective statements. This latter position is at the basis of extensive questioning and is conditional on the production of observation conditions that enable unbiased collection or, in the worst-case scenario, lead to the number of responses biased in one direction being offset by the number of those biased in the opposite direction.

   In fact, collection of information always takes place between these two determinants of the quality of what is collected—which are more or less important depending on the themes studied—and the validity of the answers will depend on the way in which the researcher is able to integrate and operate them in his solutions.

5. One of the operations that we carried out as a control on results will give us the opportunity to discuss the (in)variability of responses obtained by our questionnaire, in the course of the same time of application. Knowing already the profile of the results, which pointed to a decrease in prevalence, we found that in certain regions this decrease did not follow the general pattern, so we proceeded to apply controls to the fieldwork. To this end, we retained only those interviewees who had stated that they did not consume. This operation was justified to the surveyed population by the need to check the fieldwork, with contact made by telephone. The checks were made in three regions (the Algarve and Madeira, for alcohol consumption declarations, and the Centre region, for illicit substances declarations). For alcohol, 832 households were identified, of which 313 proved to be inaccessible for checks (37.6%). Of those that could be contacted (519) the response was maintained by 68%, while 10.4% declined to answer and 21.6% changed the sense of their answer[34]. In the case of illicit substances 1,031 households were identified, of which 415 (40.2%) could not be contacted. Of those that could be contacted (616) the initial

[34] The application carried out in 2017 confirmed these orientations.

statement was confirmed by 61.8%, with 37.7% declining to answer and 0.5% changing their statement.

Firstly, these results show us that there is a possible margin of deviation between actual and reported behaviours, although we cannot attribute all of this deviation to the validity of the questionnaire, since the justification may lie in collection errors, which are always possible and in fact are considered when calculating error margins. The fact that we detected responses that were not consistent with the expected pattern denotes that these collection errors were, in the territories where checks were carried out, higher than usual, and they were therefore corrected. What seems more significant to us, from the perspective of the relationship between individuals and the norm, is the greater flexibility of the meaning of the statement when it comes to alcohol consumption, which is culturally well accepted and so recognition of consumption poses few problems: 21.6% of individuals change their response in the case of alcohol, compared to only 0.5% who do so in the case of illicit substances. Prior to that, the number of individuals who decline to respond to the control is, for illicit substances, much higher than for alcohol: 37.7% of the individuals who could be contacted, against 10.4% for alcohol, which indicates, at the very least, greater reserve regarding the control operation.

6. Everything leads us to believe, however, that this orientation, observed in 2012, also applies to previous years. If there has been any change in the normative context, we do not know to what extent this may or may not have altered the meaning of the statements. Taking into account, however, that the validity of the questionnaire is very much based on its reliability (that is its ability to capture behaviour over time, in our case over four applications), we believe that it is demonstrated by the consistency of the trends observed in consumption statements between the first (2001) and the second application (2007) but also by the consistency observed, in general, in the reduction of prevalence observed in the 2012 application. In fact, this reduction is very uniform, since it applies to all substances licit and illicit and follows a dominant pattern: 2012 consumption

generally decreases compared to 2007 but remains above that observed in 2001. The reasons for this reduction are therefore to be found in other factors, which we shall continue to analyse[35].

Methodology and information gathering procedures: reliability

The essence of our effort to understand where we might have gone wrong focused on two other operations that served to guarantee that the methodology of the study had not been adulterated. The principle followed in the study conducted in 2012 was to strictly apply all the rules, all the procedures, all the routines of the two previous applications. However, we introduced a strategic variant, which we believe may have been at the origin of the unexpected reduction in consumption prevalence. This was the rule of no substitution of selected households that we explained above. According to this rule, selected households within the set of eligible households are not replaced in case of refusal or initial non-contact. This explains why, in previous studies, the realised sample was about 19% smaller than the planned sample. This rule forces survey staff to try as hard as possible to make contact with the household. In the 2012 application, the option was given to replace these households by other households (already previously selected[36]), after all contact possibilities have been exhausted. The reason for this orientation has to do with the contractual obligation requiring that the records of the interviews corresponding to the entire sample were submitted to the body overseeing the study. Thus, at the end of the 2012 application the sample had a total of 1,366 interviews conducted following substitution, out of a total of 6,275. The fact that, in relative terms, the number of substitutions was higher than that of cases abandoned in previous applications (about 22% versus 19%) indicates that the field teams this time decided more quickly to give up on the most difficult households. Overall,

[35] The number of households selected in each statistical section is, in principle, twice the sample size, to allow for the substitution of households that, after being contacted, are found to be ineligible.

[36] In the following applications, we opted for two different bases—with and without substitutions—maintaining the fieldwork requirements but allowing for the full implementation of the sample and the analysis of the consistency of the respective results.

households were abandoned on average after three unsuccessful attempts at contact. The interviews conducted required on average 1.9 attempts.

Analysing the profile of the responses from substitute households, we found that it is equivalent to that obtained from households interviewed without substitution. For example, lifetime prevalences of any illicit substance varied by three tenths of a percent between the two samples (with and without substitutions). This does not invalidate the fact that the rule was breached, and doubt may remain as to whether this change would justify the reduction in prevalences that occurred. We thus decided to revisit the fieldwork at the level of failures, that is households that could not be contacted and had therefore been substituted. We wanted to check whether the households most resistant to interview might have any characteristics that could bias our results. At the same time, we decided to annul all interviews done by substitution, so ensuring the full application of our methodology[37].

In addition, we decided to extend collection by implementing 20% more of the theoretical sample (estimated at 6,000 individuals), corresponding to 1,200 additional interviews, with the new households to be contacted evenly over each of the 600 statistical sections and resuming the survey sheet and the selection of households to be contacted at the point where they had been left the first time around.

Of the 1,432 new interviews planned (without replacements) 1,003 were conducted[38]. Returning to the 1,366 failed attempts allowed the recovery of 440 of these. The following table provides the breakdown of all the questionnaires applied, with the collection status and age group of interviewees. We can see that, overall, the profile of the interviewees does not change significantly, with all of them maintaining the same proximities and distances in relation to the distribution of the INE (National Statistics Institute), which we use as a reference and which determines the values of the weightings that we then proceed to apply. The most important thing, however, was to know to what extent the prevalence rates obtained from the

[37] The number of interviews not conducted is justified by household absences and refusals, individual absences and refusals, or the household not matching the chosen criteria.

[38] There is no data on permanent emigration between 2004 and 2007, nor on temporary emigration between 2004 and 2010.

initial collection, which we wanted to check, were different from those obtained with the supplementary collection, carried out in a situation of technical stress on the assumption that "something had gone wrong" in the first application. The results we obtained show that the levels of prevalence initially obtained did not change later.

Table 3-2. Comparison of real population (INE data) and populations of different segments / collection status by five-year age (unweighted data), ages 15-74, for 2012

Five-year age groups	Initial without substitutions (N=5,272)	Recovered* (N=102)	New (N=1,003)	Failed attempts (N=440)	Final total (N=6,817)	INE data
15-19	6.6	3.9	5.2	6.1	6.3	7.0
20-24	5.6	3.9	6.1	5.5	5.7	7.2
25-29	5.8	5.9	6.3	6.1	5.9	7.9
30-34	6.4	7.8	7.7	8.0	6.7	9.3
35-39	8.0	15.7	8.4	9.5	8.3	10.4
40-44	8.5	6.9	8.0	8.0	8.4	9.7
45-49	7.9	6.9	7.0	7.0	7.7	9.7
50-54	9.5	13.7	9.0	6.6	9.3	9.1
55-59	10.1	5.9	9.4	11.8	10.1	8.5
60-64	10.2	14.7	9.5	10.2	10.2	8.0
65-69	9.9	5.9	11.7	11.8	10.2	7.1
70-74	11.3	8.8	12.0	9.3	11.2	6.2
Total	100	100	100	100	100	100

*Centre, Algarve and Madeira

Reconfiguration of universe observed

From the mid-2000s onwards and as the economic and financial crisis took hold, Portugal became again a country of emigration, while the stock of immigrants decreased due to the reduction in the number of new arrivals and increase in returns. In the period between 2007 and 2012, the dates of our study, these combined movements will assume significant proportions and trigger what some indicate as constituting a demographic crisis. By targeting the "general population" our Survey could not but capture these movements and their consequences on the characteristics of the populations. Our conviction, which we now wish to discuss, is that the population we interviewed in 2007 is not the same as the one we interviewed in 2012 and that the changes that have taken place tend to affect primarily the younger population groups and males, where most of the use of psychoactive substances, especially illicit substances, is concentrated.

This hypothesis is not, however, easy to validate, since migratory flows, besides not having received constant attention by the body responsible for statistical surveys[39], may be framed within various official categories[40] between which it can be difficult to choose—between permanent and temporary migration, for example—and which bring a dimension of invisibility that is naturally associated with its at least partially clandestine dimension[41]. These circumstances open up a space of uncertainty, where estimates may be based on various different sources and classification criteria. We are interested in describing flows between 2008 and 2012 (the interval between studies) and shall rely as much as possible on official sources.

Between 2009 and 2011, the number of residence permits issued fell from 61,400 in 2009 to 50,700 in 2010, before falling further to 45,000 in 2011[42]. These permits were issued on various grounds, with the largest number (around half) being for students, and one quarter for family reunification. Only 16% were granted for work purposes[43]. The reduction in the number of new residence permits, the departure of immigrants and changes in nationality are, among other reasons, at the root of a reduction in the stock of foreign residents, which fell by about 2% in 2010 and 2011 and 4.5% in 2012 (see table below).

[39] The Organisation for Economic Co-operation and Development (OECD) refers to this difficulty in its *International Migration Outlook* (OECD, Portugal, 2013).

[40] Presenting a study on the emigration of young people to France (*Novos Emigrantes para França: a geração Europa*), João Teixeira Lopes refers to these as "invisible to institutions and to diplomacy" (Lusa news agency, 19 November 2013).

[41] Presenting a study on the emigration of young people to France (Novos Emigrantes para França: a geração Europa), João Teixeira Lopes refers to these as "invisible to institutions and to diplomacy" (Lusa news agency, 19 November 2013.

[42] OECD, Portugal, 2013, p. 286.

[43] OECD, Portugal, 2013, p. 286.

Table 3-3. Evolution of number of emigrants between 2008 and 2012

Year	Resident foreign population	% of total population
2008	440,277	1.04
2009	454,191	3.16
2010	445,262	-1.97
2011	436,822	-1.90
2012	417,042	-4.53%

Source: SEF (Immigration and Borders Service), Relatório de Imigração, Fronteiras e Asilo, 2012, p. 65.

We do not know the sociological profile of individuals who have left the category of foreigner. Without being able to enter into explanatory reasoning, we can however note that this change translates into a reduction in the prevalences of consumption in this population: the prevalence of use of any illicit psychoactive substance throughout life was 11% in 2001 among the foreign population, became 14.2% in 2007 and dropped to 9.2% in 2012.

Table 3-4. Fifetime prevalence of any psychoactive substance use, by nationality, ages 15-64, in 2001 (n=14,184), 2007 (n=12,202) and 2012 (n=5,355) (in %)

	2001	2007	2012
Total population of Portuguese nationals	7.6	11.7	9.1
Total foreign population	11.0	14.2	9.2
Total resident population	7.8	12.0	9.5

At another level, demographic developments in Portugal are also seeing a reduction in the resident population due to a new process of emigration motivated by economic reasons. According to results presented by INE[44], there were 100, 978 emigrants (permanent and temporary) in 2011 and 121,418 in 2012. Between 2008 and 2010 no data was collected. According to Jorge Malheiros[45], in the second half of the second decade of the 21st century "existing figures point to a volume (of flows) that should not be

[44] INE, *Estatísticas Demográficas*, 2012, Lisbon, 2013.
[45] Jorge Malheiros, "Portugal 2010: o retorno do país de emigração", in Janus.net, Vol. 2, n.º 1 (spring 2011), pp. 133-142,
(site observare.ual.pt/janus.net/pt_vol2_n1_not3, consulted on 15/09/13).

much below 70,000 departures per year". If this estimate is correct, we could then estimate the number of emigrants during the period at around 430,000. However, we can use known data to extrapolate the numbers for the unknown years, assuming that there are no variables that would disturb the proportionality. We thus see that in 2010 and 2011 the ratio between the number of permanent emigrants and the number of temporary emigrants is of the order of 43% to 57%. Applying this ratio to the three years for which we do not know the number of temporary emigrants, we would find a total of around 143,000 individuals, which when added to the numbers for 2011 and 2012 would give us a total of 365,000 emigrants for the period in question. Taking into account the possibility that there may be a certain number of permanent emigrants who do not appear in official counts and going by the frequent news reports about people leaving (professionals, young graduates...) this last figure could actually be an underestimate.

Based on these two estimates and considering the total population aged between 15 and 64 in 2007, we would be missing between 5.2 and 6.2% of the population in 2012. However, we know that the profile of people who emigrate is not random. The table shows that men accounted for about 70% of emigrants in 2011 and 2012 (which reflects a greater participation of women in the process, since in the previous three years, considering only permanent exits, men accounted for approximately 80% of those leaving). On the other hand, as this is economic migration, the population tends to be younger. According to Malheiros (ibidem, 140), the emigrant population "is essentially young (over 55% are under 30)". It therefore seems to us that we can consider the weight of emigrants in relation to a younger population, namely that aged between 20 and 44. In this case, the emigrant population represents between 9.6% and 11.3%, depending on whether we take a higher or lower estimate.

We believe that the replacement of 10% of the population in the groups—young and mainly male—where most consumption is concentrated is likely to significantly change the profile of the reference population. This means that the population which leaves is likely to have a sociological profile that changes the relation of these age groups with regard to consumption. More precisely, the new composition of the population of active young people has characteristics that place it at consumption levels lower than the previous similar population before emigration.

Table 3-5. Evolution of number of emigrants between 2008 and 2012

Years	Permanent emigrants			Temporary emigrants			Total emigrants		
	M	F	T	M	F	T	M	F	T
2008	16,286	4,071	20,357	--	--	--	--	--	--
2009	13,519	3,380	16,899	--	--	--	--	--	--
2010	19,008	4,752	23,760	--	--	--	--	--	--
2011	31,329	12,669	43,998	39,958	17,022	56,980	71,287	29,691	100,978
2012	34,540	17,418	51,958	53,453	16,007	69,460	87,993	33,425	121,418

Source: National Statistics Institute (INE), 2013.

One of the ways of corroborating our hypothesis consists, then, in verifying whether the average pattern of the results obtained in 2012—prevalence rates decreasing relative to 2007, but still above those observed in 2001—is verified in the age groups that feed emigration. If that is the case, there would be no reason to expect that this pattern would be observed in older age groups (for example, over 45) that are little or not at all associated with the new migratory flow. The following table shows us that this is precisely what happens: the fall in consumption is observed only in age groups up to age 44. Above this group, prevalence neither falls nor rises for the whole period between 2001 and 2012. The relatively small values of the increases between 2007 and 2012 must take into account the fact that the base of prevalences is low for these groups, especially as we move to consider older age groups.

Table 3-6. Lifetime prevalence of any illicit psychoactive substance use, by five-year age groups, ages 15-64, in 2001 (n=14,184), 2007 (n=12,202) and 2012 (n=5,355) (in %)

	2001	2007	2012
15-19	10.8	8.6	7.5
20-24	13.7	21.2	18.4
25-29	14.0	19.0	17.5
30-34	11.8	18.9	14.5
35-39	10.6	16.5	11.4
40-44	4.6	13.4	9.1
45-49	3.1	7.8	7.8
50-54	1.2	4.3	6.7
55-59	0.6	2.2	2.7
60-64	0.2	0.7	0.4
Total	7.8	12.0	9.5

Analysing the different reasons why we could have been wrong, producing an unexpected result, we can conclude that this result definitely seems to us to be associated with a change in the sociological composition of the population, following the process of emigration that took place at the time. As for other factors of a methodological nature, they will continue to occupy us, because the questions they pose will never be definitively resolved, so it will be necessary to manage them constantly. We have shown, however, that these methodological factors are not responsible for the bias observed in the cohort effect and so for the decrease in prevalence rates seen for almost all substances. We believe that the prevalence rates presented are those corresponding to the population living in Portugal at the time of application.

PART II

EVALUATION OF EFFECTS OF SURVEY TECHNIQUES ON ORIENTATION OF RESPONSES IN SURVEYS ABOUT DRUG USE IN THE GENERAL POPULATION

CHAPTER 4

PRESENTATION OF THE PROBLEM

Validity and reliability of measurements at national and international level

Surveys of the general population are important sources of information to guide policy-making regarding the use of psychoactive substances and the evaluation of their effects. It is therefore important to ensure, on the one hand, the validity of the measurements carried out that are translated into the results presented and, on the other, their reliability, that is, the ability of the instruments of measurement to apprehend their object over time. In this study we shall be more interested in the issue of validity, and consider the effect that survey techniques may have on prevalence of use.

Since the beginning of our study on the use of substances in Portugal's resident population, we opted for a survey conducted through face-to-face interviews, using the CAPI (computer-assisted personal interviewing) technique. In other countries, other techniques have been used in addition to face-to-face collection, such as interviews conducted by telephone, completion of questionnaires over the internet, or even self-completion and subsequent sending of responses by mail. These different techniques are used as alternatives, according to the choice of the respondent or the options of the research team, or in combination.

The choice of face-to-face interview was justified by the proximity of our methodology to that of studies carried out in Spain under that country's National Drug Plan, which had already built up successful experience before us, based in turn on the experience of the United States[46].

The use of psychoactive substances—licit and illicit—is a very internationalised research topic, especially since the intervention of the European Monitoring Centre for Drugs and Drug Addiction and, before that,

[46] Cf. Balsa et al. 2001.

of the Pompidou Group of the Council of Europe. However, despite the efforts to coordinate and harmonise methodologies and indicators on the part of these institutions, the truth is that the range of choices is still very heterogeneous, particularly with regard to the technical guidelines followed in the information collection phase. This heterogeneity may be justified by choices related to the survey conditions that may arise in each country (cultures in relation to consumption, availability of survey bases, penetration of means of contact such as telephone...) or by the traditions of the research teams. Finances may also be an important factor in motivating the choices that are made, since in the case of studies requiring a high number of interviews, a preference for cheaper collection techniques such as telephone interviews may be imposed, regardless of any technical considerations.

When it comes to comparing results from studies conducted using different survey techniques, we need to know to what extent these results can be effectively compared. At this point, however, we must distinguish the international from the national dimension. At the national level, in addition to the usual validity issues associated with the quality of the collection instrument, there is above all the question of the reliability of instruments of measurement over time. Indeed, regardless of the quality of the instrument of measurement, which it is hoped will be adequate, it is important to maintain it so that a change cannot alter the results obtained over time. At international level and for the purposes of comparison, the question of reliability arises, but above all that of validity, that is, the effect that the measurement technique may have on the results over the time interval chosen for the comparison. In other words, to what extent and in what sense can the collection techniques influence the orientation of the responses? This question points, on the one hand, to the limits of international comparison when different collection techniques are involved and, on the other, taking into account collection at national level, to the consequences that a change in these techniques may have on the results when trying to evaluate identical behaviour.

To account for the effects of collection techniques on the results obtained, we can follow the two paths offered by the specialised literature. At the first stage, here, we shall consider how certain circumstances associated with information collection—particularly the distance between interviewers and interviewees—can influence results across different application techniques. At a second stage, which we shall deal with in the next section, we shall focus our attention on each of the survey techniques compared here, in order to assess to what extent the distance between interviewer and interviewee can have a more or less decisive influence.

Circumstances that may influence collection results

Distance between interviewers and interviewees

One of the best known and most studied effects of collection techniques on response orientation is the presence or absence of an interviewer during the interview (De Leeuw 2005). "For sensitive or difficult questions, or questions for which socially desirable responses exist, the presence or not of a human interviewer often makes a difference in how a respondent answers." (Thompson et al. 2013, 448). This means that interviewees will tend to adjust their responses to societal norms so as not to upset the interviewer or appear deviant. But this concept of the presence of the interviewer does not distinguish between situations where the interviewer is physically present (face-to-face interviews with paper forms or using CAPI) and interviews conducted by telephone. In fact, Moskowitz (2004) and Kreuter et al. (2008), cited by Thompson (2013, 448), show that the fact that in telephone questioning the interviewer is not physically present may increase the number of socially desirable responses. The situation is, however, different in the case of answers obtained when the questionnaire is completed by the respondent, whether on the internet or before returning by post. Declarations of risk behaviours are more probable in the case of questionnaires answered online. But what seems to be at issue is the way that questions are cognitively processed by respondents (Thompson 2013).

Moreover, in the presence of an interviewer, respondents tend to simplify their response to questions containing a scale or numerical series. One possible explanation is that interviewees may feel under time pressure as the interviewer waits for them to respond. If the size of a scale is reduced, for example, interviewees spend less time positioning themselves or quantifying a particular occurrence (Kraus and Steiner 1995).

Way of presenting questions

The way in which questions are presented can also influence the accuracy of responses. This is especially true when a question has many possible responses; in this case, the accuracy of the positioning is better if the items are read by the respondent and not by the interviewer (Thompson 2013). Again, this circumstance makes it possible to distinguish situations where the interviewer is present from those where self-completion is used (internet or postal questionnaires). However, face-to-face interviews where respondents are presented with cards with response options could enhance the advantages of self-completion, although we have no information on this situation. The mode of application may also have consequences at other levels for the quality of the information collected. Thus, it has been observed that respondents choose the last two items read by the interviewer (Bishop et al. 1988, cited by Thompson 2013 and Krosnick and Alwin 1987) and that their responses focus on the two extreme positions of a Likert scale when items are read by the interviewer (Dillman et al. 2009, cited by Thompson 2013, 513, and Macer 2005); in contrast, in visual modes, respondents tend to answer closed-ended questions by positioning themselves in the first categories (Krosnick and Alwin 1987), or by using the scale more fully (Macer 2005). At the same time, respondents tend to give more positive responses to questions of scale in oral modes than in visual modes (Christian 2007).

CHAPTER 5

INSTITUTIONAL FRAMEWORK AND TECHNICAL CONDITIONS OF STUDY

Institutional framework

Since we must compare results from various sources that use different survey techniques, it is important for us to assess the effects these techniques may have on the results. The question is also important from the perspective of programming studies on behaviour that is socially condemned. In these cases, in particular, survey difficulties and the costs involved justify studying what are the most suitable solutions, to guarantee that the quality of the information will not be compromised. When, for technical reasons, the option is not to choose between several application methodologies, but to combine them in a design that integrates different approaches, it is a matter of building knowledge that makes it possible to compare the results obtained or even finding, as do M. E. Thompson et al. (2013), weighting factors that make it possible to reduce them to equivalent measurements.

Our study was carried out in conjunction with the RARHA survey[47]. The application of this study in Portugal was carried out on a representative universe of the resident population, covering the seven NUTS II regions (five in mainland Portugal and the two autonomous regions). In order to ensure the possibility of comparing the results obtained with the results of the INPG — national survey on drug use among general population, we used the same procedures in construction samples, the same techniques for selecting households and individuals, and the same survey technique: face-to-face interviews using the CAPI system.

Taking this study as the main reference, we selected 24 questions (with 51 variables), from which we built a common questionnaire to compare

[47] RARHA (Reducing Alcohol Related Harm) is a joint action on reducing alcohol-related harm, co-funded by the European Union Health Programme.

different survey techniques, limited to two mainland regions: Greater Oporto and Greater Lisbon.

When designing the questionnaire, the correct fit between the objectives of the project and the questionnaire was checked for each mode of application, and the questions that met each of the objectives were identified. A review was also made of the consistency between the questions and response categories, of the logical sequence of responses and of the filters.

A total of 589 telephone interviews were conducted using the CATI (computer-assisted telephone interviewing) system; 622 online interviews were conducted using the CAWI system (computer-assisted web interviewing) with the Intercampus panel's internet users; and 331 personal interviews were conducted using the CAPI system (computer-assisted personal interviewing).

Presentation of questionnaire

The variables considered make it possible to compare the results obtained by each of the survey techniques at the following levels: rates of prevalence of alcohol consumption, a test for alcohol abuse, and rates of prevalence of illicit psychoactive substances use, in addition to socio-demographic data that allow us to control for the effects of the survey techniques taking into account the effects that sampling techniques have on the construction of the interviewed populations.

The wording of the questions in the three versions of the questionnaire was kept as identical as possible, with only a few adaptations being made in order to respect the specificity of each of the survey techniques. Cards were used in the face-to-face questionnaire for all questions, except for those requiring dichotomous responses (yes/no) and those requiring a numerical response.

Socio-demographic characteristics

The following socio-demographic characteristics were considered in the analysis: gender, age, marital status, level of education, household size, current and/or past occupation and net monthly household income.

Consumption indicators

We selected a set of indicators of alcohol consumption from the RARHA Survey to analyse the differences in the survey modes.

In addition to a question on frequency of alcohol consumption in the last 12 months, which also allows us to calculate the prevalence of consumption, we selected the battery of questions relating to the RAPS — Rapid Alcohol Problems Screen test, to gauge problems related to this type of consumption. The test is composed of the following questions: (1) During the past 12 months have you had a feeling of guilt or remorse after drinking? (2) During the past 12 months has someone told you about things you did or said while you were drinking that you could not remember? (3) During the past 12 months have you failed to do what is normally expected of you because of drinking? and, (4) During the past 12 months did you ever have a drink first thing in the morning after waking up?

We were also interested in understanding how respondents respond in different modes when thc topic is more sensitive, involving issues such as secrecy. Thus, a block on the use of illicit psychoactive substances was included. Respondents were asked about the amount of illicit psychoactive substances—cannabis, amphetamines, ecstasy, LSD, heroin, cocaine, magic mushrooms and other substances—they had consumed in their lifetime. After this question, the respondents who declared consumption were asked to specify whether this consumption was in the last 30 days, last 12 months, or longer ago. In this way we can calculate, besides the amount of lifetime use of psychoactive substances, its prevalence in the last year and in the last month.

Presentation of collection techniques used

The process of data collection has been the subject of several studies on the advantages and disadvantages of different methodologies. The choice of method depends on a series of rather complex factors. Floyd and Fowler state that the choice of data collection mode—post, internet or personal interview—is related to the definition of the sample, the research topic, the characteristics of the sample and the availability of human resources and funds; it has implications on response rates, on the question form, and on the costs of the survey (2002, 58). Naturally, there are still other factors to be taken into account, such as the time available for collection of information, the money we can spend, and the complexity and nature of the questions, among others.

Below we present the three collection methods used for this study, describing their main characteristics, advantages and disadvantages, and the methodological and technical orientations for each one.

CATI (Computer-assisted telephone interviewing)

Presentation

In the CATI collection method, the interviewer poses the questions by telephone and records the responses on a computer.

The main advantages of this method are that it is quick, not restricted to any geographical areas so long as the population has a telephone, and technically reliable.

Among the main disadvantages is the fact that some target populations cannot be contacted. In Portugal, according to the results of the 2010/2011 IDEF, only 67.7% of the population living in Portugal had a landline; the highest proportion of households with a landline was in the Azores Autonomous Region (77.3%) and the lowest in the Algarve (59.7%). Mobile phones have a greater penetration but do not, however, allow for a representative national sample.

Two other disadvantages are the impossibility of visual observation and the difficulty of covering certain subjects that are considered to be more sensitive.

The telephone interview, by increasing the distance between respondent and inquirer, reduces the probability of obtaining responses that are socially desirable. However, it proves inadequate in cases where questionnaires are longer, as is the case with the survey on use in the general population. This reason, combined with the difficulty of building a reliable survey base from telephone directories, explains our opting for face-to-face interviews in the national survey on drug use among general population (INPG), an option that we extend to the RARHA study, under which we make this comparison, for the reasons we have stated above.

Methodological and technical orientations

The sample for the CATI application was constructed respecting a proportional distribution of the population living in the regions selected for the comparison (Greater Oporto and Greater Lisbon) and aged between 15 and 64, with quotas imposed by gender, age and territory of residence. The selection of households was carried out from public directories of landline telephone numbers. In the household the interviewee was selected from the gender and age quota matrix.

Fieldwork was carried out by Intercampus, SA and took place between 14 and 25 May 2015, conducted by 12 interviewers. All interviewers participated in training (a briefing) with interview practice.

The response rate was 61%, out of a total of 1,455 contacts made.

The following table shows the universe, the theoretical sample and the actual realised sample:

Table 5-1. CATI collection technique: universe, theoretical sample and actual sample, by gender and age groups in the Greater Oporto and Greater Lisbon regions

	UNIVERSE			THEORETICAL SAMPLE			ACTUAL SAMPLE		
	Greater Oporto	Greater Lisbon	Total	Greater Oporto	Greater Lisbon	Total	Greater Oporto	Greater Lisbon	Total
Total	882,066 (100%)	1,354,729 (100%)	2,236,795 (100%)	229 (100%)	352 (100%)	581 (100%)	231 (100%)	358 (100%)	589 (100%)
Men	424,239 (48.1%)	648,337 (47.9%)	1,072,576 (48.0%)	110 (48.0%)	168 (47.7%)	278 (47.8%)	110 (47.6%)	174 (48.6%)	284 (48.2%)
Women	457,827 (51.9%)	706,392 (52.1%)	1,164,219 (52.0%)	119 (52.0%)	184 (52.3%)	303 (52.2%)	121 (52.4%)	184 (51.4%)	305 (51.8%)
15-24	139,623 (15.8%)	214,820 (15.9%)	354,443 (15.8%)	36 (15.7%)	56 (15.9%)	92 (15.8%)	36 (15.6%)	56 (15.6%)	92 (15.6%)
25-34	178,350 (20.2%)	296,017 (21.9%)	474,367 (21.2%)	46 (20.1%)	77 (21.9%)	123 (21.2%)	47 (20.3%)	83 (23.2%)	130 (22.1%)
35-44	203,139 (23.0%)	317,901 (23.5%)	521,040 (23.3%)	53 (23.1%)	82 (23.3%)	135 (23.2%)	53 (22.9%)	82 (22.9%)	135 (22.9%)
45-54	192,867 (21.9%)	271,435 (20.0%)	464,302 (20.8%)	50 (21.8%)	71 (20.2%)	121 (20.8%)	50 (21.6%)	71 (19.8%)	121 (20.5%)
55-64	168,087 (19.1%)	254,556 (18.8%)	422,643 (18.9%)	44 (19.2%)	66 (18.8%)	110 (18.9%)	45 (19.5%)	66 (18.4%)	111 (18.8%)

Source: INE — National Statistics Institute — Data for the population resident in the areas of Greater Oporto and Greater Lisbon at the time of the 2022 Census, aged between 15 and 64, Recenseamento da população e habitação — Censos 2011, and Relatório técnico, Intercampus.

For this application a quality control exercise was carried out using the following operations:

1. As the information was collected via the CATI system, the data file was automatically validated at two levels: validation of the response codes, question by question, and a validation of the interaction between questions (skips and filters), while respecting the structure of the questionnaire used.
2. During collection, direct supervision of the work of interviewers was carried out in loco. This work was thus always monitored by an Intercampus field technician, who ensured compliance with instructions with regard to the method of selecting interviewees, and also checked the conditions in which the interview was carried out and its duration.

CAWI (Computer-assisted web interviewing)

Presentation

In the CAWI collection method, the questionnaire appears in the browser as a web page that respondents can access in different ways, depending on the sample design. The computerised environment enables a great deal of logical complexity in the interviewing process. Filters and the application of logical relations determine that only the questions to be answered appear on the screen. Questionnaire responses are immediately recorded on the server, allowing the collection of information and the results to be monitored on an ongoing basis. This technique allows multimedia materials (images, speech recordings or music files) to be integrated into the questionnaire, although this was not the case with our study.

The main advantages are: 1) no printing, interviewer or data recording costs; 2) collection time can be reduced; 3) information processing is done in real time; 4) easier access to certain populations (internet users, active population...); 5) there are no restrictions in access to territories, so long as they are covered by the network; 6) biases due to the presence of an interviewer are no longer observed; 7) possible errors on the part of the interviewer and in recording information are eliminated; 8) respondents have all the time they need to ponder possible responses or carefully read all the positions on a scale, without fear of delaying an interviewer; 9) finally, this survey medium, by allowing the respondent to control the process, also has the advantage of increasing confidence in anonymity.

As for disadvantages, the use of CAWI 1) may constitute an obstacle in populations unfamiliar with this type of technology; 2) does not admit of building a representative sample of the national population: according to IDEF findings (INE 2012), in 2010/2011 a computer was available in 57.2% of households nationally, and in 2012, according to Eurostat data[48], 61% of households had internet access; the elderly are one of the groups underrepresented here; 3) there are also difficulties in verifying the validity of the responses and the identity of the respondent; 4) the greater ease of giving up filling out the form increases the risk of a higher rate of incomplete questionnaires; finally, 5) an application with CAWI brings the obligation to guarantee the protection of individual data.

Methodological and technical orientations

Application of the questionnaire with CAWI was aimed at achieving a representative sample of the resident population of the regions of Greater Oporto and Greater Lisbon, considering gender and age (between 15 and 64).

The questionnaires were carried out with a panel of internet users set up by Intercampus, SA in 2009, based on invitations to respondents to the company's quantitative studies, and which currently has around 6,000 panellists nationally. Fieldwork took place between 18 and 25 May 2015. The response rate was 33% out of a total of 1,885 invitations sent out with a direct link to the website where the questionnaire was hosted.

The following table presents information on the distribution of the universe of the sample actually obtained.

---

[48] Study measuring proportion of dwellings with one or more inhabitants aged between 16 and 74 that have internet access. http://ec.europa.eu/eurostat/statistics-explained/index.php/Information_society_statistics_-_households_and_individuals/pt_households_and_individuals/pt

Table 5-2. CAWI collection technique: universe, theoretical sample and actual sample, by gender and age groups in the Greater Oporto and Greater Lisbon regions

	UNIVERSE			THEORETICAL SAMPLE			ACTUAL SAMPLE		
	Greater Oporto	Greater Lisbon	Total	Greater Oporto	Greater Lisbon	Total	Greater Oporto	Greater Lisbon	Total
Total	882,066 (100%)	1,354,729 (100%)	2,236,795 (100%)	229 (100%)	352 (100%)	581 (100%)	251 (100%)	371 (100%)	622 (100%)
Men	424,239 (48.1%)	648,337 (47.9%)	1,072,576 (48.0%)	110 (48.0%)	168 (47.7%)	278 (47.8%)	116 (46.2%)	168 (45.3%)	284 (45.7%)
Women	457,827 (51.9%)	706,392 (52.1%)	1,164,219 (52.0%)	119 (52.0%)	184 (52.3%)	303 (52.2%)	135 (53.8%)	203 (54.7%)	338 (54.3%)
15-24	139,623 (15.8%)	214,820 (15.9%)	354,443 (15.8%)	36 (15.7%)	56 (15.9%)	92 (15.8%)	43 (17.1%)	59 (15.9%)	102 (16.4%)
25-34	178,350 (20.2%)	296,017 (21.9%)	474,367 (21.2%)	46 (20.1%)	77 (21.9%)	123 (21.2%)	59 (23.5%)	90 (24.3%)	149 (24.0%)
35-44	203,139 (23.0%)	317,901 (23.5%)	521,040 (23.3%)	53 (23.1%)	82 (23.3%)	135 (23.2%)	55 (21.9%)	85 (22.9%)	140 (22.5%)
45-54	192,867 (21.9%)	271,435 (20.0%)	464,302 (20.8%)	50 (21.8%)	71 (20.2%)	121 (20.8%)	50 (19.9%)	71 (19.1%)	121 (19.5%)
55-64	168,087 (19.1%)	254,556 (18.8%)	422,643 (18.9%)	44 (19.2%)	66 (18.8%)	110 (18.9%)	44 (17.5%)	66 (17.8%)	110 (17.7%)

Source: INE — National Statistics Institute – Data for population resident in the Greater Oporto and Greater Lisbon areas at the time of the 2011 Census, aged between 15 and 64, Recenseamento da população e habitação — Censos 2011, and Relatório técnico, Intercampus.

All panel procedures comply with ESOMAR and ISO 20 252 standards, with the following quality controls:

- registration carried out in two stages, with authentication link,
- removal of duplicate registrations,
- quarantine periods, in order to avoid professional respondents,
- use of individual links for responses, with tracking of respondents.

As the information was collected through the CAWI system, the data file was automatically validated at two levels: validation of the response codes, question by question, and a validation of the interaction between questions (skips and filters), while respecting the structure of the questionnaire used.

CAPI (Computer-assisted personal interviewing)

Presentation

In the CAPI collection method, the interviewer uses a computer screen to read the questions and inserts the responses into it.

The main advantages of this method are: 1) better management of the face-to-face interview process, avoiding the use of paper and allowing better control of filters; 2) better display of materials (cards with response modalities, for example, can be shown to the interviewee); 3) recording of responses directly in the database; and 4) better and faster control of interviewers' work.

The main disadvantage of CAPI is its high cost.

Methodological and technical orientations

In the RAHRA study we followed the same methodology used in the national survey on drug use among general population (INPG), to ensure the possibility of comparison between the two studies. The sample results from a draw in multiple stages, stratified by conglomerates, with the selection of primary units (municipalities) and secondary units (statistical sections), in a random and proportional way. The selection of the final units of observation—households—is carried out randomly on the basis of a prior survey of the dwellings that exist in the sections and, within the household, the choice of the individual to be interviewed is made by drawing lots using tables of numbers that are also random.

In case of refusal on the part of the selected individual or in cases (duly attested) of absence from the home, substitutions are not allowed to be made through any technique applied by the interviewee or by the team in charge on the ground, with these individuals replaced from the list of substitutes that resulted from the same draw that guarantees the random character of the sample that serves for the first selection.

For the purposes of this methodological comparison study, the interviews conducted in the Greater Lisbon and Greater Oporto regions were selected from the sample drawn for the RARHA study (the national population living in mainland Portugal and the autonomous regions and aged between 15 and 64, in both cases inclusive).

The table below presents the history of contacts made and their results:

Table 5-3. CAPI collection technique: record of contacts made and results (n)

Contacts established	**608**
Not selectable	173
Outside universe (not eligible)	81
Outside quota	14
Individual absent	78
Interview requested	435
Refusal by household	53
Refusal by individual	42
Interview conducted (valid)	331
Other situations	9
Interview conducted, not valid	(7)
Incomplete interview	(2)
Contacts not established due to household absence	**52**
Total households visited	**660**

Source: Technical report, Intercampus.

In cases of refusal, we considered two types of situations:

- Refusal by the selected individual — when the person in the household who was selected declines to answer the questionnaire.

- Refusal by the household — when the interviewer does not get to select the person to be surveyed, because someone in the household declines the questionnaire.

Absence of contact is counted when the following situations occur:

- Absence of persons in the household — after successive contacts at different times of the day, the household is reported as uncontactable.
- Absence of the selected individual — after having been selected, the person to be interviewed is never found and, for this reason, no interview takes place.
- Impossible to access the household — in some, not very frequent cases, some households that were part of the sample could not be contacted, for different reasons: doormen who did not allow access, the existence of dogs guarding access, etc.
- Other situations — cases not previously identified, but which for some reason should not be included in the analysis. Despite the initial exhaustive survey of these situations, there are however cases that it was not possible to identify in the first phase, such as uninhabited homes, offices or individuals who do not fit the criteria defined for the survey population.

The response rate is 58.2% (while for the sample actually obtained nationally it was 61%).

Table 5-4. CAPI collection technique: universe and actual sample, by gender and age groups in the Greater Oporto and Greater Lisbon regions

	UNIVERSE			ACTUAL SAMPLE		
	Greater Oporto	Greater Lisbon	Total	Greater Oporto	Greater Lisbon	Total
Total	875,584 (100%)	1,344,179 (100%)	2,219,763 (100%)	118 (100%)	213 (100%)	331 (100%)
Men	420,562 (48.0%)	642,957 (47.8%)	1,063,519 (47.9%)	64 (54.2%)	107 (50.2%)	171 (51.7%)
Women	455,022 (52.0%)	701,222 (52.2%)	1,156,244 (52.1%)	54 (45.8%)	106 (49.8%)	160 (48.3%)
15-24	138,152 (15.8%)	211,862 (15.8%)	350,014 (15.8%)	13 (11.0%)	32 (15.0%)	45 (13.6%)
25-34	172,172 (19.7%)	285,316 (21.2%)	457,488 (20.6%)	12 (10.2%)	34 (16.0%)	46 (13.9%)
35-44	202,521 (23.1%)	320,678 (23.9%)	523,199 (23.6%)	28 (23.7%)	56 (26.3%)	84 (25.4%)
45-54	193,456 (22.1%)	273,026 (20.3%)	466,482 (21.0%)	21 (17.8%)	47 (22.1%)	68 (20.5%)
55-64	169,283 (19.3%)	253,297 (18.8%)	422,580 (19.0%)	44 (37.3%)	44 (20.7%)	88 (26.6%)

Source: INE — National Statistics Institute — Data for population resident in Greater Oporto and Greater Lisbon areas, aged between 15 and 64, Resident population (N. º) by Place of residence (NUTS — 2013), Sex and Age group; Annual, Annual estimates of resident population, 2015, and Technical report, Intercampus.

CHAPTER 6

INFLUENCE OF COLLECTION TECHNIQUES ON CONSTRUCTION OF OBSERVED POPULATIONS

Response rates

Many researchers have analysed the factors likely to influence response rates. Analysis by Steeh (1981), for example, shows that there is a substantial increase in non-response due mainly to refusal by respondents. Her results also reveal that these trends are related to the degree of urbanisation: the higher the urbanisation, the higher the refusal rates. It is of interest to consider this relationship in our test since it focused on the Greater Oporto and Greater Lisbon areas, where trends of increasing urbanisation are observed. Given data for the study carried out using face-to-face interviews for RARHA at the national level, we can indeed observe that the response rate at the national level is higher (61%) than the one observed in the test (58%).

When we consider survey techniques, the experience reported in the scientific literature indicates that online surveys obtain rather modest response rates (Fricker and Schonlau 2002; S. Fricker et al. 2005). Our results allow us to state that the physical presence of or even just contact with an interviewer increases the probability of participation of the surveyed population. Comparing the three data collection methods used, the CAWI method had the lowest response rate, at 33%, while the collection techniques in which an interviewer was involved resulted in higher response rates: 58% with CAPI and 61% with CATI.

Table 6-1. Sample size and response rate by information collection method

	CAPI (Computer-assisted personal interviewing)	CATI (Computer-assisted telephone interviewing)	CAWI (Computer-assisted web interviewing)
Sample size	331	589	622
Response rate	58%	61%	33%

Source: Technical reports, Intercampus.

Construction of populations observed by survey technique

Although all the techniques tested seek to build a representative sample of the population, respondents end up presenting slightly different socio-demographic characteristics depending on the survey method: CAPI, CATI or CAWI. The following table shows the breakdown of the populations by gender and 10-year age groups, before any weighting is carried out. We shall analyse them first, since they are characteristics (along with the distribution of the interviews over the territory) that enter into the construction of the theoretical samples that are the basis of any survey technique. We shall then analyse other characteristics (marital status, level of education, etc.) that, while not interfering in the construction of the sample, will present a distribution more in line with the universe insofar as the sample that produced them is representative of this same universe.

To this end, we shall compare the results obtained in each of the three samples with the INE data or, in their absence, with the data from the national survey on drug use among general population, Portugal 2016/17 (INPG). The latter, besides the date of application being close to the date of application of the three test samples, presents data representative of the national population — its universe being the population living in mainland Portugal and in the Autonomous Regions of Madeira and Azores, aged between 15 and 64.

Table 6-2. Distribution of samples by gender and age groups by information collection method

	Universe		CAPI		CATI		CAWI	
	n	%	n	%	n	%	n	%
Total	2,219,763	100	331	100	589	100	622	100
Gender								
Men	1,063,519	47.9	171	51.7	284	48.2	284	45.7
Women	1,156,244	52.1	160	48.3	305	51.8	338	54.3
10-year age groups								
15-24	350,014	15.8	45	13.6	92	15.6	102	16.4
25-34	457,488	20.6	46	13.9	130	22.1	149	24.0
35-44	523,199	23.6	84	25.4	135	22.9	140	22.5
45-54	466,482	21.0	68	20.5	121	20.5	121	19.5
55-64	422,580	19.0	88	26.6	111	18.8	110	17.7

Source: INE — National Statistics Institute and Databases of national survey on drug use among general population, Portugal (INPG).

a) Gender

When considering respondents' gender, CATI collection (M: 48.2% / W: 51.8%) shows the best approximation to the distribution of the universe (M: 47.9% / W: 52.1%). This approximation is mainly due to the fact that with the CATI application it is possible to control the characteristics of the sample taken, by defining quotas. This control is impossible in the case of CAWI to the extent that, once the panel is mobilised to access the platform, whoever wants to respond does so. Women (54.3%) thus appear to be more willing than men (45.7%) to answer. In the case of CAPI, since it is a representative sample in which the statistical sections, households and respondents are selected randomly, the characteristics of the universe are in principle progressively achieved at the level of larger territorial units, but not necessarily immediately and at the level of small territorial units. Although the two territorial units are sufficiently large for the gender breakdown to align, this does not happen, with proportions between men and women inverting (M: 51.7% / W: 48.3%) compared to the theoretical sample (M: 47.9% / W: 52.1%). This distortion is thus due to difficulties in achieving the sample in the field that are associated with the survey technique itself and particularly the strict protocol that we followed. It is likely that these factors reinforce each other, and they are further corroborated by the already reported increased rate in refusals to respond to this type of approach.

b) Age groups

The analysis orientations that we presented for gender are also valid for age groups, another variable that allows the stratification of the theoretical samples. Once again, there is a greater control of ages with CATI, with age being one of the quotas defined to select the individuals: any possible bias that may occur during the collection process will have to be rectified at some point by restoring the missing groups to the sample. The CATI sample is therefore closer to the distribution observed at the level of the universe, with relatively small deviations and no clear pattern: an overrepresentation of the 25-34 age group is offset by small under-representations of all the others. The same is not true for the CAWI sample. Online collection shows a clear overrepresentation of the 25-34 age group and an underrepresentation of the individuals aged 35 and over. We can thus generalise and say that CAWI underrepresents older groups and overrepresents the younger ones, since the 15-24 age group is also overrepresented, but not as much as the 25-34 age group. With regard to the sample conducted through the CAPI, we observe a clear underrepresentation of the youngest groups, especially the 25-34 age group, and a very clear overrepresentation of the 55-64 age group. Once again, this distortion is due to the difficulties in applying the techniques for selecting individuals on the ground, with this being aggravated when substitutions are not allowed in the event of a refusal to respond.

c) Civil status

When we consider civil status, there is a greater approximation to the universe in the CAPI sample with regard to the widow(er) category, and in the CATI and CAWI samples with regard to the married or cohabiting and single categories. The weight of divorced persons is uniform in the three samples and similar to the universe.

Table 6-3. Sociodemographic data in different samples: civil status

	INPG DATA 2016/17* n=2,322		CAPI n=331		CATI n=589		CAWI n=622	
	n	%	n	%	n	%	n	%
Married or non-marital partnership	1,166	50.2	193	58.3	315	53.4	333	53.6
Single	831	35.8	92	27.8	218	37.0	231	37.1
Divorced	232	10.0	26	7.9	46	7.8	48	7.7
Widow(er)	83	3.6	16	4.8	5	0.8	8	1.3
No response	9	0.4	4	1.2	5	0.8	2	0.3

* Greater Lisbon & Greater Oporto

Source: Databases of national survey on drug use among general population, Portugal (INPG).

d) Educational level

It is collection by the CAPI technique that presents the best approximation to the distribution of the universe, regardless of the level of education considered. The CATI and CAWI samples have twice as many or more respondents with higher education. Online studies using panels tend to have samples with more informed individuals than samples in face-to-face studies (Duffy, Smith, Terhanian and Bremer 2005). Smith et al. (2013) find that there is greater participation of individuals with a higher level of education in online questionnaires, but that this factor does not affect the response behaviour of participants.

Table 6-4. Sociodemographic data in different samples: educational level

	INPG DATA 2016/17* n=2,322		CAPI n=331		CATI n=589		CAWI n=622	
	n	%	n	%	n	%	n	%
Below primary	48	2.1	4	1.2	3	0.5	1	0.2
Basic 1st cycle	261	11.2	50	15.1	40	6.8	7	1.1
Basic 2nd & 3rd cycles	853	36.7	94	28.4	80	13.6	51	8.2
Secondary	529	22.8	102	30.8	188	31.9	192	30.9
Vocational/Post -secondary	16	0.7	2	0.6	14	2.4	32	5.1
Higher	419	18.0	73	22.0	257	43.6	338	54.4
Not specified	--	--	1	0.3	1	0.2	0	0.0
No response	196	8.4	5	1.5	6	1.0	1	0.2

* Greater Lisbon & Greater Oporto

Source: Databases of national survey on drug use among general population, Portugal (INPG).

e) Employed population

On the question of whether the person interviewed was in work at the time of the interview, the CAPI sample (58.9%) shows the best approximation to the distribution of the universe (53.2%). The CAWI sample has the highest percentage of people in work (71.4%).

Table 6-5. Sociodemographic data in different samples: current employed population

	DATA 2016/17* n=2,322		CAPI n=331		CATI n=589		CAWI n=622	
	n	%	n	%	n	%	n	%
Yes	1,236	53.2	195	58.9	372	63.2	444	71.4
No	896	38.6	135	40.8	208	35.3	174	28.0
No response	190	8.2	1	0.3	9	1.5	4	0.6

* Greater Lisbon & Greater Oporto

Source: Databases of national survey on drug use among general population, Portugal (INPG).

f) Household size

Where household size is concerned, it is the CAPI sample that, once more, allows a closer approximation with the universe. The CAWI and CATI samples present a higher percentage of non-responses to this question.

Table 6-6. Sociodemographic data in different samples: household size

	DATA 2016/17* n=2,322		CAPI n=331		CATI) n=589		CAWI n=622	
	n	%	n	%	n	%	n	%
Lives alone	360	15.5	57	17.2	64	10.9	80	12.9
2	739	31.8	111	33.5	150	25.5	155	24.9
3	695	29.9	87	26.3	171	29.0	181	29.1
4	412	17.7	52	15.7	133	22.6	136	21.9
5 or more	116	4.9	24	7.2	46	7.6	86	8.0
No response	0	0.0	0	0.0	25	4.2	20	3.2

* Greater Lisbon & Greater Oporto

Source: Databases of national survey on drug use among general population, Portugal (INPG).

Influence of survey techniques on consumption declarations

Results obtained before any weighting

Now that we know that the three collection methods tend to build relatively different survey populations, we shall see how they differ when it comes to observing consumption behaviour. We will proceed to an analysis of the results obtained from each of the three samples, initially without adding any weighting, that is, focusing on a reading on the influence of the modes of collection. We shall take as reference data the results of the national survey on drug use among the general population (INPG), conducted by us in 2016/17 — the only study of the three that presents representative data of the national population (limited here just to the 18 municipalities of Greater Lisbon and Greater Oporto that participated in the test)[49].

In any case, the results of the test interest us less for the (obviously limited) information they provide on the prevalence of use than for the opportunity to compare the results obtained through the three applications.

Consumption of alcoholic beverages

Lifetime and last-year abstainers are more often captured by CAPI than by CATI and CAWI, which record more "weekend users" (consumption between 1 and 2 days a week). But the latter two modes of collection also more often record users with other weekly frequencies (between 3 and 4 days, but especially between 5 and 6 days) or more sporadic consumption. The distance from the interviewer thus seems to facilitate consumption declarations. The exception is the lower presence of daily consumption in the CAWI technique.

---

[49] We do not exclude the possibility that some of the divergences found may be due to slight differences in the wording of the questions between the INPG questionnaire and that of the RARHA, the study under which the test was conducted.

Table 6-7. Consumption in different samples: frequency of last-year consumption of alcoholic beverages

	DATA 2016/17* n=2,322		CAPI n=331		CATI n=589		CAWI n=622	
	n	%	n	%	n	%	n	%
Every day	383	16.5	47	14.2	86	14.6	62	10.0
5 to 6 days a week	55	2.4	19	5.7	52	8.8	71	11.4
3 to 4 days a week	107	4.6	16	4.8	34	5.8	35	5.6
1 to 2 days a week	320	13.8	56	16.9	129	21.9	182	29.3
2 to 3 days a month	161	6.9	23	6.9	52	8.8	44	7.1
Once a month	91	3.9	15	4.5	38	6.5	37	5.9
6 to 11 days a year	77	3.3	14	4.2	44	7.5	48	7.7
2 to 5 days a year	119	5.1	36	10.9	63	10.7	67	10.8
Once a year	34	1.5	11	3.3	20	3.4	13	2.1
No drink in last year but drank before	621	26.8	51	15.4	22	3.7	21	3.4
Has never drunk alcohol	341	14.7	43	13.0	49	8.3	40	6.4
No response	13	0.6	--	--	--	--	--	--

* Greater Lisbon & Greater Oporto

Source: Databases of national survey on drug use in the general population, Portugal (INPG).

When we consider the indicators of harmful consumption summarised in the RAPS test questions[50], this orientation is maintained: it is in the CAWI sample that the percentages of affirmative responses to the four items are higher. In this case, there are no marked differences between the samples applied in CAPI and CATI.

[50] The four questions that make up the RAPS test are only put to those who said they drank at least between 6 and 11 times a year. As for the INPG questions, they have different wording and response modalities from those used in the RARHA questionnaire. In the INPG, the four indicators used here, which make up the RAPS test, correspond to questions 5 to 8 of the AUDIT test.

Table 6-8. Consumption in different samples: indicators of RAPS test

	DATA 2016/17* n=2322		CAPI n=331		CATI n=589		CAWI n=622	
	n	%	n	%	n	%	n	%
Feelings of guilt or remorse								
Yes	27	1.2	8	2.4	19	3.2	40	6.4
No	295	12.7	179	54.1	414	70.3	430	69.1
No response	--	--	3	0.9	1	0.2	1	0.2
Not applicable	--	--	0	0.0	1	0.2	10	1.6
Missing system	2,000	86.1	141	42.6	154	26.1	141	22.7
Someone has told them about things they did or said while drinking that they do not remember								
Yes	26	1.1	14	4.2	27	4.6	55	8.8
No	296	12.8	173	52.3	399	67.7	406	65.3
No response	--	--	3	0.9	0	0.0	1	0.2
Not applicable	--	--	0	0.0	9	1.5	19	3.1
Missing system	2,000	86.1	141	42.6	154	26.1	141	22.7
Has failed to do what is normally expected of them due to drinking								
Yes	16	0.7	10	3.0	13	2.2	38	6.1
No	307	13.2	177	53.5	416	70.6	428	68.8
No response	--	--	3	0.9	0	0.0	2	0.3
Not applicable	--	--	0	0.0	6	1.0	13	2.1
Missing system	2,000	86.1	141	42.6	154	26.1	141	22.7
Has a drink first thing in the morning after waking								
Yes	10	0.4	3	0.9	4	0.7	8	1.3
No	313	13.5	184	55.6	430	73.0	467	75.1
No response	--	--	3	0.9	0	0.0	2	0.3
Not applicable	--	--	0	0.0	1	0.2	4	0.6
Missing system	2,000	86.1	141	42.6	154	26.1	141	22.7

* Greater Lisbon & Greater Oporto

Source: Databases of national survey on drug use in the general population, Portugal (INPG).

Use of illicit psychoactive substances

More than in the case of alcohol, the questioning about the use of illicit substances imposes the reasons that the respondent would have to censor their behaviour in the presence of an interviewer.

In fact, it is among respondents in CAPI that the prevalence of the use of illicit psychoactive substances is lower. Not only do fewer people say they consume, regardless of the time period considered (lifetime, last year or last month), but among those who said they consumed, they are the ones who consumed the least substances and the ones who did so the least often.

It is in CAWI, where the distance between interviewee and interviewer is greater, that appear the highest prevalence of use and the largest number of substances consumed a greater number of times.

Table 6-9. Consumption in different samples: questions about illicit substances

	DATA 2016/17* n=2,322		CAPI n=331		CATI n=589		CAWI n=622	
	n	%	n	%	n	%	n	%
Number of times cannabis consumed								
1 to 5 times	100	4.3	8	2.4	71	12.1	101	16.2
6 or more times	98	4.2	19	5.7	84	14.3	117	18.8
Never	2,002	86.2	284	85.8	434	73.7	404	65.0
Don't know/No response	122	5.2	0	0.0	0	0.0	0	0.0
Missing system	0	0.0	20	6.0	0	0.0	0	0.0
Number of times amphetamines consumed								
1 to 5 times	9	0.4	3	0.9	10	1.7	25	4.0
6 or more times	2	0.1	2	0.6	6	1.0	8	1.3
Never	2,309	99.4	306	92.4	573	97.3	589	94.7
Don't know/No response	3	0.1	0	0.0	0	0.0	0	0.0
Missing system	0	0.0	20	6.0	0	0.0	0	0.0
Number of times ecstasy consumed								
1 to 5 times	11	0.5	3	0.9	7	1.2	12	1.9
6 or more times	5	0.2	1	0.3	6	1.0	11	1.8
Never	2,299	99.0	307	92.7	576	97.8	599	96.3
Don't know/No response	7	0.3	0	0.0	0	0.0	0	0.0
Missing system	0	0.0	20	6.0	0	0.0	0	0.0

Number of times LSD consumed								
1 to 5 times	7	0.3	3	0.9	9	1.5	16	2.6
6 or more times	2	0.1	3	0.9	4	0.7	6	1.0
Never	2,309	99.4	305	92.1	576	97.8	600	96.5
Don't know/No response	4	0.2	0	0.0	0	0.0	0	0.0
Missing system	0	0.0	20	6.0	0	0.0	0	0.0
Number of times heroin consumed								
1 to 5 times	4	0.2	2	0.6	6	1.0	8	1.3
6 or more times	1	0.0	2	0.6	5	0.8	7	1.1
Never	2,303	99.2	307	92.7	578	98.1	607	97.6
Don't know/No response	14	0.6	0	0.0	0	0.0	0	0.0
Missing system	0	0.0	20	6.0	0	0.0	0	0.0
Number of times cocaine consumed								
1 to 5 times	16	0.7	2	0.6	8	1.4	17	2.7
6 or more times	4	0.2	3	0.9	16	2.7	19	3.1
Never	2,280	98.2	306	92.4	565	95.9	586	94.2
Don't know/No response	23	1.0	0	0.0	0	0.0	0	0.0
Missing system	0	0.0	20	6.0	0	0.0	0	0.0
Number of times magic mushrooms consumed								
1 to 5 times	9	0.4	3	0.9	8	1.4	15	2.4
6 or more times	0	0.0	0	0.0	2	0.3	3	0.5
Never	2,313	99.6	308	93.1	579	98.3	604	97.1
Don't know/No response	0	0.0	0	0.0	0	0.0	0	0.0
Missing system	0	0.0	20	6.0	0	0.0	0	0.0

* Greater Lisbon & Greater Oporto

Source: Databases of national survey on drug use among general population, Portugal (INPG).

When we consider statements on lifetime prevalence of the use of illicit psychoactive substances, it is the CAPI sample that is closest to the universe, which is not surprising because the two results were constructed using identical techniques.

Table 6-10. Consumption in different samples: prevalence of use of illicit substances

	DATA 2016/17* n=2322		CAPI n=331		CATI n=589		CAWI n=622	
	n	%	n	%	n	%	n	%
Lifetime consumption prevalence								
Any substance**	334	14.4	28	8.5	159	27.0	223	35.9
Cannabis	320	13.8	27	8.2	155	26.3	218	35.0
Cocaine	42	1.8	5	1.5	24	4.1	36	5.8
Amphetamines	13	0.6	5	1.5	16	2.7	33	5.3
Ecstasy	23	1.0	4	1.2	13	2.2	23	3.7
Heroin	19	0.8	4	1.2	11	1.9	15	2.4
LSD	13	0.6	6	1.8	13	2.2	22	3.5
Magic mushrooms	9	0.4	3	0.9	10	1.7	18	2.9
Last-year consumption prevalence								
Any substance**	152	6.5	13	3.9	39	6.6	57	9.2
Cannabis	144	6.2	11	3.3	38	6.5	54	8.7
Cocaine	11	0.5	1	0.3	4	0.7	10	1.6
Amphetamines	13	0.6	0	0.0	2	0.3	6	1.0
Ecstasy	5	0.2	1	0.3	0	0.0	3	0.5
Heroin	2	0.1	2	0.6	0	0.0	3	0.5
LSD	2	0.1	3	0.9	1	0.2	4	0.6
Magic mushrooms	0	0.0	0	0.0	0	0.0	3	0.5
Last-month consumption prevalence								
Any substance**	120	5.2	8	2.5	20	3.4	22	3.5
Cannabis	117	5.1	7	2.1	20	3.4	22	3.5
Cocaine	4	0.2	0	0.0	1	0.2	2	0.3
Amphetamines	0	0.0	0	0.0	1	0.2	1	0.2
Ecstasy	1	0.0	0	0.0	0	0.0	2	0.3
Heroin	1	0.0	1	0.3	0	0.0	1	0.2
LSD	0	0.0	0	0.0	0	0.0	1	0.2
Magic mushrooms	0	0.0	0	0.0	0	0.0	0	0.0

* Greater Lisbon & Greater Oporto

** Other substances mentioned by respondents include: incense sold in smart shops, lavender, opium, MD, MDMA, spider poppers/spray.

Source: Databases of national survey on drug use among general population, Portugal (INPG).

We sought to construct an indicator that would allow us to synthesise this different information and, at the same time, establish some hierarchy in the relationships found. We chose to perform a logistic regression between the different intervening variables, organising a model where the variable to be explained is the existence or not of a declaration of consumption. We used two separate pieces of information: one concerning the lifetime prevalence of the use of illicit psychoactive substances, and another concerning the frequency of consumption of alcoholic beverages.

Regarding the variables likely to influence the consumption statements we considered, on the one hand, the individual characteristics of respondents (gender, age group and, in a second stage of the analysis, level of education) and, on the other, the three survey modes. We isolated the effect of the concomitant variables in order to assess the individual effect of each one. These variables will be analysed as predictors of reported consumption.

Overall, the results of this analysis point to a significant predictive ability of the different intervening factors, even if the percentage of variance explained is relatively low.

We confirmed that affirmative statements regarding the use of illicit psychoactive substances are associated with personal characteristics: gender (with a predominance of men) and age (with emphasis on the 25-34 age group).

We also confirmed that the survey mode, after controlling for the effect of interviewees' individual characteristics, is another predictor: the chances of declaring consumption are significantly lower in CAPI mode and higher in CAWI mode.

The influence of education levels, when included in the model, is not statistically significant.

Table 6-11. Odds ratio of predictors of declarations of lifetime use of illicit substances

PREDICTIVE VARIABLES	Use of illicit substances	
	Model 1 **Odds ratio**	**Model 2** **Odds ratio**
Gender	Cat. ref.: Women	Cat. ref.: Women
Men	1.527 (1.193-1.954)*	1.567 (1.220-2.013)**
Age groups	Cat. ref.: 55-64	Cat. ref.: 55-64
15-24	1.911 (1.231-2.968)*	1.754 (1.118-2.751)*
25-34	3.082 (2.047-4.640)**	2.617 (1.709-4.006)**
35-44	2.405 (1.615-3.580)**	2.098 (1.390-3.167)**
45-54	2.079 (1.380-3.132)**	1.956 (1.291-2.963)**
Survey modes	Cat. ref.: CATI	Cat. ref.: CATI
CAPI	0.253 (0.164-0.390)**	0.280 (0.181-0.434)**
CAWI	1.509 (1.177 1.933)*	1.441 (1.22-1.852)**
Educational level		Cat. ref.: Medium
Lower		0.706 (0.475-1.049)
Higher		1.186 (0.907-1.558)
	$\chi^2(7)=133.940$**	$\chi^2(9)=140.932$**

Odds ratio and 95% confidence interval for the association between lifetime use and personal variables and survey mode (and, in the second model, level of education).
Model 1: R2CS=0.083; R2N=0.121 / Model 2: R2CS=0.087; R2N=0.127
* p<0.05, ** p<0.001
Source: Databases of national survey on drug use among general population, Portugal (INPG).

We followed the same procedures to analyse the statements on alcohol consumption. However, instead of dichotomising the positions between users or non- users, we chose to introduce into the model information on the frequency of consumption, considering five positions—'daily/almost daily', 'weekly', 'monthly', 'less often' or 'never'—using a multinominal logistic regression. We thus differentiated not only the occurrence or non-occurrence of reporting consumption, but also the regularity with which consumption occurs. We used the previous explanatory model, having included in a second stage of the analysis educational level as a predictive variable.

Both the individual characteristics considered and the mode of enquiry continue to be predictive of reported consumption. Taking the category of no consumption ('never') as a benchmark, and looking at the characteristics of individuals, we observe that: 1) the probability of reporting more frequent consumption is higher in men; 2) the probability of reporting daily consumption is lower for the 15-24 and 25-34 age groups; and 3) weekly consumption is more frequent in the 25-34 and 35- 44 age groups. After controlling for the effect that individual characteristics may have on statements, we also found that responses vary according to the survey mode: the probability of reporting daily, weekly, monthly or less frequent consumption is higher in CATI and CAWI, compared to the CAPI benchmark. In this case, education appears as a differentiating factor in the consumption of beverages, with the minimum level of compulsory education corresponding to a reduction in the reported frequency of consumption.

Table 6-12. Odds ratio of predictors of declarations of lifetime consumption of alcoholic beverages

FREQUENCY OF CONSUMPTION	PREDICTIVE VARIABLES	Alcohol consumption	
		Model 1 Odds ratio	Model 2 Odds ratio
Daily/almost daily	**Gender**	Cat. ref.: Women	Cat. ref.: Women
	Men	6.150**	6.553**
	Age groups	Cat. ref.: 55-64	Cat. ref.: 55-64
	15-24	0.076**	0.065**
	25-34	0.485*	0.355**
	35-44	0.729	0.551*
	45-54	1.076	0.910

	Survey mode	Cat. ref.: CATI	Cat. ref.: CATI
	CAPI	3.127**	2.590**
	CAWI	3.953**	3.187**
	Educational level		Cat. ref.: Higher
	Lower		0.515*
	Higher		0.879
Weekly	**Gender**	Cat. ref.: Women	Cat. ref.: Women
	Men	3.070**	3.493**
	Age groups	Cat. ref.: 55-64	Cat. ref.: 55-64
	15-24	1.269	0.796
	25-34	2.473*	1.278
	35-44	2.334*	1.309
	45-54	1.565	1.154
	Survey mode	Cat. ref.: CATI	Cat. ref.: CATI
	CAPI	3.101**	2.118**
	CAWI	4.952**	2.873**
	Educational level		Cat. ref.: Higher
	Lower		0.171**
	Higher		0.657
Monthly	**Gender**	Cat. ref.: Women	Cat. ref.: Women
	Men	1.620*	1.828*
	Age groups	Cat. ref.: 55-64	Cat. ref.: 55-64
	15-24	2.328*	1.471
	25-34	2.984*	1.624
	35-44	2.885*	1.685
	45-54	1.670	1.252
	Survey mode	Cat. ref.: CATI	Cat. ref.: CATI
	CAPI	2.967**	2.142*
	CAWI	3.130**	2.171*
	Educational level		Cat. ref.: Higher
	Lower		0.222**
	Higher		0.712
Less frequently	**Gender**	Cat. ref.: Women	Cat. ref.: Women
	Men	1.147	1.243
	Age groups	Cat. ref.: 55-64	Cat. ref.: 55-64
	15-24	1.683	1.171
	25-34	2.841**	1.885*
	35-44	2.371*	1.600
	45-54	1.553	1.246
	Survey mode	Cat. ref.: CATI	Cat. ref.: CATI
	CAPI	2.519**	2.018*
	CAWI	2.965**	2.171*

Educational level		**Cat. ref.: Higher**
Lower		0.411**
Higher		0.919
	$\chi^2(28)$=414.536**	$\chi^2(36)$=460.468**

Odds ratio and 95% confidence interval for the association between lifetime use and personal variables and mode of enquiry.
Model 1: R2CS=0.236; R2N=0.247; R2MF=0.086; Model 2: R2CS=0.260; R2N=0,272; R2MF=0.096
* $p<0.05$, ** $p<0.001$
Source: Databases of national survey on drug use among general population, Portugal (INPG).

These results allow us to conclude that: 1) the mode of enquiry makes the orientation of the consumption declaration vary; 2) after controlling for the effect of the characterisation variables, the orientation of the consumption declaration is different according to the lawfulness of the substance, with a higher propensity to declare alcohol consumption in face-to-face collection mode and a higher propensity to declare use of illicit substances when the survey is carried out online or on the telephone.

Weighted results

The data we have just analysed relate to unweighted results because these are the only way of directly measuring the deviations that each collection technique imposes on the data. Weighting them would, in the first place, correct in the CAPI sample the distortions that we introduced when we decided not to fully respect the proportionality of the weight of the population in the regions. But a second type of correction that a weighting can make to the three samples is justified by the small distortions that may occur during the sample planning and collection operations. The errors in the programming of the sample result from the fact that the questionnaires were distributed to the regions taking into account a breakdown of the estimated population.

This correction is of interest, above all, from the perspective of obtaining a more accurate knowledge of behaviours, which is not what we are aiming at here. For this reason, we shall not detail these results, which are dealt with in other studies. We are, however, interested in highlighting the bias that the survey techniques have on the construction of the survey populations and, consequently, on the results obtained: when we correct the samples on the basis of the control variables (gender, age and region of residence) we are not able to obtain in the CATI and CAWI samples a correction at the level of other individual characteristics of the population, as is the case, for example, with education levels. This is achieved after applying the weighting to our reference sample and the CAPI collection technique.

Final considerations

The main conclusion that we can draw from our analysis is to underscore the differences in the results obtained when different collection techniques are used.

At the beginning of this century François Beck and P. Peretti-Watel, in a study of youth consumption, found that "when the questions asked deal with 'sensitive' topics, the mode of collection seems to have an impact on the answers obtained" — a conclusion that according to the authors may not apply to some types of survey, namely general population surveys (Beck and Peretti-Watel 2001). The solution proposed by the authors is to test collection techniques that can eliminate biases, so guaranteeing reliable responses, if possible.

In the same period Winter (1999), in a comparative study promoted by the European Monitoring Centre for Drugs and Drug Addiction, applied a survey on the prevalence of use among general population using three different methods (postal, telephone and face-to-face) in three European countries (the Netherlands, Greece and Sweden). In view of the diversity of results, the authors prefer to relativise the effect of the collection methods, concluding that the type of method used does not matter much, as it will only imply small differences in the results obtained. Far more important as a source of error, according to them, is the issue of non-response, as it is often linked to specific groups. The use of different methods implies a greater variety of distortions; however, there is reason to believe that their effect will be less important than that caused by non-response. As this is considered to be the main problem, the research team recommends that different survey methods be applied simultaneously, as in that way distortions resulting from the types of non-response induced by each of the methods can be corrected.

The design and implementation of mixed modes of application thus began to be proposed at the beginning of this century as a response to the various problems presented by each method when applied in isolation. The literature shows that higher response rates can be obtained by using mixed modes (Duffy, Smith, Terhanian and Bremer 2005). However, we know that different collection techniques lead to different results. The challenge identified since the beginning of the century has not yet been overcome, two decades later. However, many works have been devoted to tackling it.

François Beck, who has done important research in the field of drug studies and particularly in general population surveys, has dedicated the past dozen years to developing multi-mode collection methods, and currently heads the programme at INSEE (Institut National de la Statistique et des Études Économiques). The 2019 INSEE report presents multi-mode collection as the technique of the future for collecting statistical information from households (INSEE 2019, 45).

In Portugal, the National Statistics Institute (INE) is advancing on the same path of multi-mode collection, introducing collection via the internet, namely in its census operation (see, in particular, INE 2017, 125 and 127).

Multi-mode techniques involve collection via self-completed online questionnaires (CAWI), replacing the classical face-to-face collection. The internet is presented as a complementary technique for households that are comfortable with this methodology. However, it does not substitute the participation, when necessary, of an interviewer, who may use various approaches, usually the telephone (CATI). Furthermore, the methodology benefits from a structure offering support for completion (Ibidem, 48).

In parallel with the construction of multi-mode collection platforms, statistical techniques are developed to correct any distortions associated with each of the techniques used.

PART III

SCALES AND MEASURES OF ALCOHOL CONSUMPTION IN THE GENERAL POPULATION

Introduction

Epidemiological knowledge of alcohol consumption, of patterns and volumes, of acute and chronic consequences, and of the determining factors is of particular importance for the planning of public policy. Monitoring alcohol consumption in a population is crucial for assessing whether national policies and approaches are effective in reducing alcohol-related problems (WHO 2010; WHO 2012). As we read in the latest *Global Status Report on Alcohol and Health*, "Local, national and international monitoring and surveillance frameworks are needed to monitor the magnitude and trends of alcohol consumption and related harm, as well as to monitor policy responses in conjunction with analysis of trends in alcohol consumption and alcohol-attributable disease burden." (WHO 2018, 28).

However, estimating alcohol consumption by individuals and societies is complex and difficult. To measure the levels of alcohol consumption in the population, we can use direct measures (based, for example, on sales of alcohol beverages) and/or indirect measures (based on data collected from the population). Both direct and indirect measures have advantages and disadvantages that need to be understood. It is of interest to reflect on methodological problems, different organisational and service cultures and even different cultural models that make it difficult to obtain quantified and comparable estimates of the prevalence and incidence of consumption and its patterns, associated problems and determining factors across different studies.

In this section we seek to clarify in how the issue of measuring the amount of alcohol consumed in Portugal has been addressed. In the first chapter we shall address the importance of monitoring alcohol consumption, discussing the guidelines of direct and indirect measures and their advantages and disadvantages. We shall review best international practice regarding the measurement of alcohol consumption, focusing—with no pretensions of exhaustiveness—on international studies and guides that discuss problems of definition and measurement of population-based consumption, namely estimates of per capita consumption. In the next chapter we shall present the main sources of data on alcohol consumption in Portugal using global and national statistical sources, sources in the alcoholic beverage industry, public health compendia and databases, and population-based studies. We shall confront global and national statistics relating to production or public health data with the results of the two most recent population-based studies we conducted: the RARHA SEAS 2015 and the INPG 2016/17.

CHAPTER 7

MONITORING OF CONSUMPTION

Measuring alcohol consumption

Measuring is an integral part of our daily lives: we routinely classify and assign values to people and objects without much reflection on the processes underlying our decisions and assessments. In the sciences, notably statistics and epidemiology, the ranking and ordering of values must be done systematically, and there are clear rules for developing different types of measures, and criteria to decide which are most appropriate to answer a specific research question (Weisburd and Britt 2014).

While estimating alcohol consumption by individuals and societies is difficult, the epidemiology of alcohol consumption and its related problems plays a vital role in monitoring consumption patterns in populations.

As we shall see in more detail below, levels of alcohol consumption can be measured using various indicators, the most important and commonly used being prevalence (or the number) of current alcohol consumers or abstainers, total per capita alcohol consumption in litres of pure alcohol per person per year, and alcohol consumption in grams of pure alcohol per person per day (WHO 2018).

According to the World Health Organization, the two main ways to collect information on alcohol consumption in a population are alcohol sales data and general population surveys (WHO 2000).

Direct measures of levels of alcohol consumption include sales data, or information that allows for a more precise estimate of the amount of alcohol consumed by the population in a given year. Governments regularly monitor sales data for tax collection purposes, and these figures may be collected from government publications or agencies.

While annual sales data are often very accurate, they may not necessarily reflect consumption, as beverages purchased in a given year may not be consumed in that same year (notably with respect to premium and/or aged wines — although these products generally constitute only a small portion of total consumption). Furthermore, alcohol vendors may increase their stock in anticipation of a tax increase, which may artificially distort the data (Kling 1991). These figures also do not take into account unrecorded alcohol (Lachenmeier, Gmel and Rehm 2013), namely domestic production, alcohol smuggled across borders, and illegal production (Rehm 2014; Moskalewicz, Room and Thom 2016). According to Manthey and colleagues, unrecorded alcohol accounted for about 25% of global alcohol consumption in 2017 (2019, 2494).

As for indirect measures, data on individual alcohol consumption obtained through general population surveys have advantages over other measures such as sales data. They measure not only volume but also individual consumption patterns (WHO 2000); in this way, researchers can link consumption to problems arising from it or, rather, adjust the characteristics of consumption to the individual level (Dawson 2003), allowing for comparison of consumption drinking patterns between population subgroups (WHO 2000). Another advantage of survey data is the possibility of describing patterns and volume of consumption. Data on consumption patterns are needed to measure the volume or proportion of alcohol consumed at high-risk levels.

Other main strengths of general population surveys include probabilistic random sampling, which allows generalisation to the whole population; the use of samples to capture the largest possible segment of the total population; and the ability to calculate the margins of error with which results are presented.

One of the disadvantages of surveys, as mentioned in some studies, is their underestimation of alcohol consumption: estimated consumption usually represents only 30%-60% of total alcohol sales (Moskalewicz, Room and Thom 2016; Bellis et al. 2009; Boniface and Shelton 2013; WHO 2018). This underestimation is mainly due to sampling problems (Shield and Rehm 2012), bias due to non-responses (Gorman et al. 2014) and underreporting bias (Livingston and Callinan 2015). Thus, although population surveys are powerful epidemiological tools we must bear in mind, in addition to the drawbacks mentioned above, that they do not present exact consumption, but rather consumption as self-reported by respondents; moreover, they almost always exclude significant population groups, such as the homeless or institutionalised populations, among others (Adlaf 2005).

We shall deal with all these aspects in more detail in the following chapters.

International recommendations for measuring alcohol consumption

We now proceed to a non-exhaustive survey of international guidelines that offer recommendations for measuring alcohol consumption. We shall first present the guidelines and studies that outline these recommendations and then attempt to systematise them.

Guides and studies

International Guide for Monitoring Alcohol Consumption and Related Harm | World Health Organization

This guide was developed by the World Health Organization 20 years ago to provide guidance on epidemiological monitoring of alcohol consumption and to improve the global and regional comparability of data on alcohol use and alcohol-related problems (WHO 2000). Written by a large number of experts on alcohol (WHO 2000, i), this guide is structured in four parts: I) Introduction; II) Measurement of alcohol volume and consumption patterns (with reflections on the estimation of per capita alcohol consumption, estimates of alcohol consumption levels and patterns with the use of national surveys, and other methodological issues on monitoring alcohol consumption); III) Measures and indicators of alcohol-related problems (namely, problems relating to health, police and other official statistical sources; problems mainly attributable to long-term alcohol use; and harm mainly attributable to the acute or short-term effects of alcohol consumption); and IV) Summary and recommendations.

Agreement on ways to measure alcohol consumption | Kettil Bruun Society (KBS)

A conference with the theme of social and epidemiological research on alcohol consumption was stated by the Kettil Bruun Society (KBS) from 3 to 7 April 2000 in Skarpö, Sweden, attended by more than 40 researchers from 12 countries with a tradition of research in this area. The conference aims were to develop a possible consensus around methods of measurement and analysis in alcohol surveys. The results were summarised by Deborah A. Dawson and Robin Room in the article "Towards agreement on ways to measure and report drinking patterns and alcohol-related problems in adult general population surveys: the Skarpö Conference overview" (Dawson and Robin 2000).

Recommended Alcohol Questions | National Institute on Alcohol Abuse and Alcoholism (NIAAA)

In 2003, a working group of the National Institute on Alcohol Abuse and Alcoholism (NIAAA, 2003) met in Bethesda, Maryland, United States to develop recommendations on a minimum set of questions regarding alcohol consumption, for questionnaires that include a limited number of questions on the subject.

Standardizing Measurement of Alcohol-Related Troubles (SMART) | European Commission

The SMART project, funded by the European Commission, published its guidelines and recommended alcohol questions for European countries in 2010. This project developed standardised methodologies for comparative research in the European Union on excessive consumption, episodic heavy consumption/binge drinking, context of consumption, alcohol dependence and alcohol-related problems, unrecorded alcohol, self-harm and harm caused by third-party consumption, and attitudes towards alcohol policies (Moskalewicz and Sieroslawski 2010). The methodology, developed on the basis of a review of European research experiences in more than 20 countries as well as a review of the literature, was tested in 10 countries with different sociocultural backgrounds and consumption patterns.

Reducing Alcohol Related Harm (RARHA) | European Union

The Joint Action on Reducing Alcohol Related Harm (RARHA 2016) was a joint action submitted by Portugal, coordinated by its General Directorate for Intervention on Addictive Behaviours and Dependencies (SICAD), and included in the European Union's Second Programme of Community Action in the Field of Health. Aiming to support action in reducing alcohol-related harm, it involved 28 member states plus Iceland, Norway and Switzerland, and a number of partners, associates and collaborators, including public entities, several NGOs and international organisations such as the OECD, WHO, EMCDDA and the Pompidou Group.

This joint action consisted of six work packages. WP4 — Monitoring — was led by Poland (PARPA), with Germany (IFT) as co-leader. The NOVA University of Lisbon – School of Social Sciences and Humanities (NOVA FCSH) — CESNOVA, in coordination with SICAD, took part in this work package. WP4 aimed to strengthen the methodology for research on harmful alcohol consumption and the comparative analysis of consumption patterns and associated harm in all member states, developing a standardised monitoring approach in order to establish a basis for comparative assessment and monitoring of trends. WP4 was followed up in two ways: 1) RARHA SEAS (Standardised European Alcohol Survey) — production of a common survey for all member states to obtain comparable data regarding consumption (Computer patterns in these countries; 2) RARHA HARMES (Harmonising Alcohol-Related Measures in Europe) — comparison of results from existing alcohol-related surveys in member states.

In RARHA SEAS a total of 33,291 interviews of respondents aged 18-64 from 19 countries were conducted. The following areas were covered in the questionnaire: sociodemographic characteristics, binge drinking, consumption contexts, unrecorded alcohol, reasons for consumption and non-consumption, attitudes towards alcohol policies, impact of others' consumption, and prevalence of problems (RAPS).

How and what to measure

The recommendations from the guides and studies mentioned above emphasise that surveys measuring alcohol consumption need to include items on average consumption volume and frequency and volume of excessive alcohol consumption, calculated by multiplying the quantity and frequency of occasions of relevant consumption in the last year.

A minimum set of three questions (which can be used to obtain all of the above measures of alcohol consumption) are provided by the guidelines: last-year and lifetime consumption status/prevalence; last-year consumption volume; and last-year frequency and volume of excessive consumption.

Beyond this minimum, the studies outline recommended items for surveys that might include a larger number of questions. To measure the average volume of alcohol consumption, questions on Beverage-Specific Quantity Frequency (BSQF) were identified as the most appropriate survey instrument, while quantity-frequency (QF) questions were identified as appropriate when resources are limited. This method is based on only two questions—“how much alcohol do you usually drink?” and “how often do you drink?”—and is recommended to be used only if limited space is available in a national survey, for example one on more general topics.

All guidelines recommend questions using the graded quantity-frequency (GQF or GF) method to assess heavy episodic drinking. This is a cost-effective method that can ensure that most of the essential information is gathered in eight questions. GQF questions start by asking for the highest level of consumption on any occasion in the last year and then, based on the response, come a series of follow-up questions about frequency of underage drinking (Dawson and Room 2000; World Health Organization 2000; Moskalewicz and Sierosławski 2010; Moskalewicz, Room and Thom 2016). The SMART and RARHA studies recommend this method because it provides the highest estimates of annual consumption and offers reliable predictions of problems related to the alcohol consumption, and most respondents find it relatively easy to answer (Sierosławski 2011).

The review of literature undertaken in the SMART study confirmed that the approach based on frequency of consumption of a specific amount of an alcoholic beverage (Beverage Specific Quantity Frequency — BSQF) works well in international comparative research (Bloomfield, Hope and Kraus 2013). Moreover, it is the approach most frequently used in Europe to measure alcohol consumption, according to the analysis conducted of 27 European countries as part of the SMART study (Sierosławski, Foster and Moskalewicz 2013).

The BSQF measure employs questions about the frequency of consumption of certain types of alcoholic beverages over a defined period and the respective quantities usually consumed on the same occasion (consumption episode) or in a day.

The advantages of using this measure as a European standard are as follows:

1. The questions in the questionnaire are understandable even for respondents with lower intellectual abilities;
2. The wording of the questions is in line with respondents' everyday experiences and consistent with the way respondents think;
3. Alcohol-related behaviours are reported in a straightforward way, not requiring any complicated calculations or other operations from respondents;
4. Only six questions are used, so implementation is not time-consuming;
5. The method captures key variations in consumption cultures, including beverage preferences.

The BSQF measure does have its limitations. Two of its shortcomings are that it cannot capture variations between different types of alcoholic beverages consumed on the same occasion or estimate the overall frequency of consumption when each beverage is asked about separately. Furthermore, the average amount of alcohol consumed per occasion, or per day, cannot be estimated because we do not know how often a respondent consumes a combination of various types of alcoholic beverages in that period of time.

As complementary information, there is the method of generic quantity/frequency, which can indicate the generic frequency of alcohol consumption and the average amount of alcohol consumed per occasion or day. However, it has two serious shortcomings. First, it fails to capture variations in different consumption cultures associated with different alcoholic beverages. Second, it forces respondents to recalculate drinking practices that may differ on a standard quantitative measure—a "standard drink"—something that is generally difficult for them, especially for those who drink multiple alcoholic beverages and are unfamiliar with the concept of a "standard drink". Moreover, in this approach, respondents may report only the beverage that is most typical for their regular consumption pattern, and not consider beverages that they consume irregularly. The "standard drink", which emerged in the United States (Bloomfield, Hope and Kraus 2013), takes into account a variety of alcoholic beverages with very different alcohol content, usually consumed in glasses of different volumes, and is used to help consumers measure their own alcohol consumption. However, as the volume of alcohol in a drink also differs and the test is still new or unknown in various consumption cultures, its application as a comparable measure is not feasible in European comparative studies.

While in epidemiological studies levels of consumption are usually expressed in grams of pure alcohol, in consumption guidelines communicated to the public, grams are often translated into "standard drinks" or "units", which are supposedly more practicable to quantify the amount of alcohol consumed. According to the results of RARHA WP5 (Montonen 2016), the content in grams of pure alcohol varies between European Union countries, with a modal value of 10 grams and a convergence towards an average of 11 grams.

There are different time references in the questions on alcohol consumption, the most common being 12 months, although 30 days and seven days are also used. There are difficulties with all of these time references. It is likely that many respondents will have difficulty remembering how they drank over a 12-month period. However, the 30- or seven-day approach fails to capture irregular seasonal drinking patterns and, of course, those who have only abstained from drinking in the last month or week (Dawson 2003). It is important to bear in mind that the "last 30 days" period is not necessarily representative of the whole year due to seasonal variation.

Most surveys ask participants to estimate their alcohol consumption with reference to one day, although some use the term "one occasion". The reference "one occasion" presents some problems, as it is very imprecise in terms of duration (how long does an occasion last?) and representation: how representative is an "occasion" as a typical form of drinking? "One day" is more easily understood and defined and has therefore been adopted as a standard time period in questions about the volume of alcohol consumed.

Questions on consumption context are also recommended by all studies that ask whether or not participants drank at mealtimes, alone or with others, and the place of consumption. Additional measures of alcohol consumption have been recommended in some of the studies; for example, the WHO, as well as SMART and RARHA, recommends including questions on unrecorded alcohol.

As for the type of alcoholic beverages, there is an extremely wide range. These drinks are present in almost all societies, the most common being wine, whose alcoholic volume generally ranges from 10% to 14%; beer, in which it can vary from 0.5% to 14%; and spirits, which can contain more than 35% pure alcohol.

Beer is available in almost all countries and much of it comes from transnational producers, their subsidiaries, joint ventures or local partners. There is a wide variety of beers, including low-alcohol or non-alcoholic; stronger still beers and other malt-based products can reach up to 14% alcohol. Brewers have created many variants: iced, dry, light, white, black, etc. Most beers contain between 4% and 6% alcohol.

Table 7-1. Some brands, types, volume and alcohol percentage of beers sold in Portugal

Brand	Type	Volume (cl)	Alcohol (% vol.)
Sagres[51]		33	5.0
Sagres	Preta	33	4.1
Sagres	Radler Limão	33	2.0
Sagres	Bohemia Original	33	6.2
Sagres	Bohemia Trigo	33	6.0
Sagres	Bohemia Puro Malte	33	7.0
Sagres	Cascade	20	4.9
Super Bock[52]		20, 25, 33 e 50	5.2
Super Bock	Stout	20, 25 e 33	5.0
Super Bock	Abadia	33	6.4
Super Bock	Coruja – American Amber Lager	33	5.3
Super Bock	Coruja – India Pale Ale Ipa	33	6.0
Super Bock	Coruja – Hoppy Lager	33	4.5
Super Bock	Green	20 e 33	2.0
Sovina[53]	Stout	33 e 75	5.2
Sovina	Trigo	33 e 75	4.9
Sovina	Amber	33	6.0
Sovina	Bock	33	7.5
Sovina	Lager	33	5.2
Sovina	Ipa	33	6.0

Spirits vary greatly in alcohol percentage, as the distillation process can produce liquids with very high alcohol content. Distillates with more than

[51] Source: http://www.sagres.pt/pt/produtos/
[52] Source: https://www.superbock.pt/pt/pt/products/
[53] Portugal's first craft beer.
Source: https://cervejartesanal.com/produtos/
For more information see, for example,
https://cervejaartesanalportuguesa.pt/cervejas/

50% alcohol are rare in international trade, but local products with this percentage of alcohol where present in informal economies may pose health risks. Some local spirit varieties do not appear in the figures recorded by international sources because they are often produced for domestic consumption or in the informal economy. They are thus not captured in tax, retail sales or industrial goods reports.

Wines generally range in strength from 10% to 14% alcohol. Grape-based products with high alcohol content, such as sherries, ports and brandies, are generally classified as distilled beverages, although the alcohol content can be as low as 20%. Informal wine production, from grapes or other raw materials, is extremely difficult to measure. Even in countries with a tradition of production, such as France, only rough estimates can be obtained of the amount of wine that, because it is made for home consumption, does not appear in official figures.

Table 7-2. Some brands, types, volumes and alcohol percentage of wines sold in Portugal

Name	Volume (cl)	Alcohol (% vol.)
Vinha de Mazouco Reserva, Região Demarcada do Douro[54]	75	14.5
Monte Sacro Branco	37.5 and 75	12.1
Planura, vinho Regional Alentejano	37.5 and 75	13.7
Tulipa	75	15.0
2017 Casal da Fradissa tinto Trás-os-Montes[55]	75	14.0
2017 Quinta da Atela Reserva tinto, Tejo	75	14.5
2018 Monte da Carochinha Rosé, Península de setúbal	75	13.0
2016 Júlio Bastos Dona Maria tinto, Alentejo	75	14.0
Bolota Alentejana, vinho tinto regional alentejano[56]	75	15.0
Bolota Alentejana, vinho branco regional alentejano	75	13.0
Real Fundação	75	14.0
Port wine (there is huge diversity with a set of designations making it possible to identify the different types of port).[57]		Between 19 and 22

[54] Source of information for the first four wines in the table: https://www.superbockgroup.com/

[55] Source of information for this and following wines in the table: https://www.garrafeiranacional.com/vinho.html

[56] Source: http://www.vinhosvm.com/vinhos-regionais-bolota.html

[57] Source: http://www.winesofportugal.info/pagina.php?codNode=18091

At the end of the 20th century, the range of alcoholic beverages could be divided into two categories: global commodities and local products. Within these two categories, there is wide variation. The global commodity category encompasses those alcoholic beverages present in international trade, tending to fall into three main categories: beer made from barley, wine from grapes, and distilled spirits.

Data from the United Nations Food and Agriculture Organization (FAO) indicate that production of alcoholic beverages has grown steadily worldwide since 1970. However, this growth has not been equivalent between categories: while the production of beer and distilled beverages has increased, the production of wine has, in general, decreased.

Finally, a standard drink unit is a simplified way of measuring the volume of pure alcohol in an alcoholic beverage and is used in many countries to guide and facilitate the calculation of daily or weekly intake. Although drinks contain different amounts of alcohol, the different types and sizes of glasses mean that the amount of alcohol ingested is about the same, which corresponds to 10 to 12 grams of alcohol per glass/cup or one standard drink unit.

Figure 7-1. Standard drink unit

	Beer	Wine	Aperitif	Brandy
Volume of glass	3 dl	1.65 dl	0.5 dl	0.5 dl
Pure alcohol content	12 g	12 to 13 g	10 to 12 g	14 to 16 g

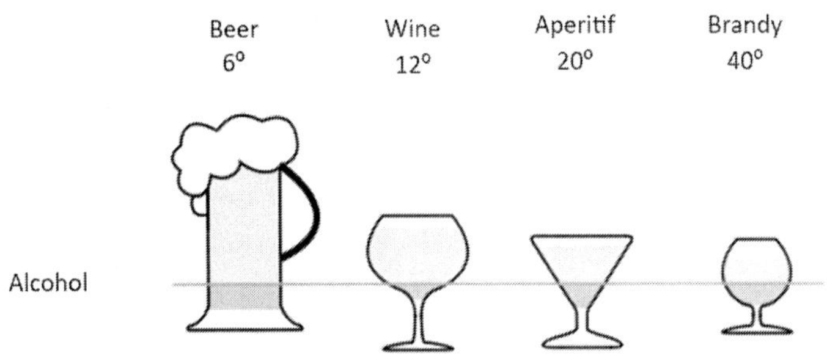

Source: Figure from Maria Lucília Mercês de Mello; José Carvalho Barrias; João Joaquim Breda, 2001, *Álcool e Problemas Ligados ao Álcool em Portugal* (Lisbon: Direcção-Geral da Saúde, 19).

Problems of definition and measurement in population-based studies

The main aim of population-based studies investigating alcohol consumption is to obtain valid and accurate measures of consumption that contribute to our knowledge and can be used to inform public policy. Full achievement of this goal depends partly on the interaction between sampling methods used, interview mode and the nature of the study population (Adlaf 2014).

Let us look at some of the challenges posed by definition and measurement in surveys of the general population.

Technical and methodological aspects

Given their contexts, objectives and dimensions, many of the studies collect information on alcohol consumption either as part of surveys on the use of psychoactive substances (e.g. National survey on drug use among general population — INPG 2001, 2007, 2012, 2016/17), or in health surveys (e.g. National Health Survey 1987, 1995/1996, 1998/1999, 2005/2006, 2014 and 2019). Other studies exist in which the contextualisation problem is alcohol itself (RARHA). All these studies focus on the general population, which means that they do not previously select their target populations according to any relationship with the consumption studied. They aim to measure the prevalence and incidence of substance use and to determine the factors associated with it, which as we noted earlier can be considered in quite different ways according to the disciplinary orientation or study problem adopted by the authors.

As for the definition of the universe of study, although there is a concern to promote universes of study that enable international comparison of the results obtained, this goal is not always achieved. Taking into account the fact that consumption behaviours are very much associated with the age of individuals, studies carried out based on different cohorts will hardly be comparable. For this reason, as mentioned in the comparative study of the European Monitoring Centre for Drugs and Drug Addiction (EMCDDA 1997), the age of the respondents is one of the criteria most generally considered when defining the universes of study. Despite the efforts made to achieve comparable results, the minimum and maximum age limits of the individuals interviewed vary substantially from one study to another.

Comparisons may also be hindered by the different treatment given to certain characteristics of the populations, such as nationality, military service status, the types of residence units selected (individual or collective, e.g. hospitals, treatment centres, prisons, barracks...), the inclusion or not of "homeless" populations, foreign residents (the language of the questionnaire may lead to the exclusion of foreigners), among others. There is also the possibility of weighting certain population groups according to the importance they may have for the study.

Regarding sample characteristics, the choice of a precise framework should be carefully evaluated to avoid any possible bias. For example, household surveys exclude segments of the population (homeless individuals, those in institutions, military personnel, etc.) who may account for a certain proportion of alcohol consumption in a country. With regard to the methodological principles underlying the definition of the samples used to carry out the studies, there is a diversity of experiences regarding their size, the observation units considered (individuals or aggregates), planned levels of representativity, the quality of the survey base, and the way in which the survey population is constructed. Sampling procedures are highly dependent on the population lists available (central population registers, files made up from postcodes, telephone lists, etc.). Other alternatives exist, as in the case of the INPG (Balsa et al. 2003, 2008, 2014, 2018), where random selection of households is carried out within sample points (statistical sections) selected in turn in an equally random manner over the entire national territory (cf. details below). The sampling method that is most appropriate for calculating the prevalence of use in the general population is, as we have seen, the probabilistic sample, both because of the possibility of controlling sampling error and consequently of determining the margin of error and confidence intervals, and because of the large number of individuals that it is usually necessary to interview in this type of sample.

The questionnaire application methods used in consumer research are also quite varied. Survey questioning mediated by computer systems in which it is the respondent who operates these systems offer the advantage of increasing trust in anonymity but may be an obstacle in populations unfamiliar with this type of technology. With regard to telephone interviews, although this situation increases the distance between respondent and interviewer and may favour trust for the type of survey to be carried out, it proves to be a factor of inefficiency in longer interviews. Procedures such as questionnaires sent by post have been occasionally put into practice, but in the perception of the respondent, they appear to jeopardise anonymity. Trust in the anonymity of responses can be further enhanced by mixed procedures.

Levels and patterns of alcohol consumption

A critical factor that will affect the approach used to measure alcohol consumption in surveys is the length of the reference period, that is, the length of time during which the respondent is asked to describe their consumption.

The inclusion of prevalence measures of alcohol consumption varies greatly from survey to survey. Often only lifetime consumption prevalence is measured, sometimes only prevalence in the last year and/or last month, and sometimes prevalence in the last week. The determining factors for the choice of one of these prevalence measures seem to be the survey context and objectives. Some surveys on psychoactive substances use the same measures of lifetime, last-year and last-month prevalence for illicit substances as recommended by the European Monitoring Centre for Drugs and Drug Addiction to measure the prevalence of licit substances (this is the case for the INPG). In health surveys, the inclusion of prevalence indicators tends to be more limited. In most countries where national health surveys measure the prevalence of alcohol consumption, only the last-year prevalence measure is used. Some experts choose not to use lifetime prevalence of alcohol consumption as they do not consider it a meaningful indicator since abstinence from alcohol consumption is quite low. The EMCDDA proposes in its "model questionnaire" measures of lifetime and last-month prevalence of alcohol consumption, while the WHO proposes the measure of prevalence of consumption in the last year or, when there is an opportunity to increase the number of alcohol questions in questionnaires, both lifetime and last-year prevalence measures. As for frequency of consumption, this is preferably the last year and the last month, but countries that conduct alcohol surveys ask about the last seven days, and the WHO also uses seven days. According to WHO, the "last seven days" indicator of frequency of consumption gives the possibility of so-called exact recall.

This method, which is based on collecting the frequency and amount of consumption on each of the seven days preceding the interview, has the disadvantage of making it impossible to verify consumption over longer periods. One of the advantages lies in the identification of habitual consumers and intensive consumption, instead of characterising lifetime consumption. When asked about usual consumption over a certain period of time (usually long), respondents tend to minimise abusive consumption. Another disadvantage of using the seven-day time frame is that it is quite sensitive to the period during which the questionnaire is administered and may over- or underestimate consumption prevalence. Hence the alternative indicator "frequency of consumption in the last week". To get around the issue of respondents having abstained in the week before the questionnaire was administered, the question was changed to last week in which consumed (not necessarily in the week before the survey was administered). In most surveys, frequency of alcohol consumption is measured by the number of days in the last year, the number of times in the last month, or the average frequency in the last month. Some countries distinguish between weekdays and weekend days.

As for the indicator "consumption quantity", fewer studies use it. Portugal's national health surveys measure the amount of alcohol consumed in the last week. A large number of countries use one or two questions to measure binge drinking over a certain period of time. In most European countries, binge drinking is defined as consuming six or more glasses on the same occasion. Another question that arises in relation to indicators of prevalence and patterns of alcohol consumption is their quantification by day or by occasion. In countries where alcohol consumption occurs mainly at mealtimes, the number of drinks consumed per day has a different interpretation from the type of consumption that occurs only on one occasion. The solution lies in asking about the amount of consumption per occasion rather than the amount consumed per day. Generally, national health surveys quantify consumption by occasion. This is the case in Portugal's national health surveys (1987 and 1995/1996) where questions are asked about the amount of wine, beer, *bagaço* (marc)/brandy, port/vermouth/liqueurs and whisky/gin consumed with lunch, snacks, dinner and other occasions.

A large proportion of the questionnaires analysed chose to discriminate the type of beverage in indicators of prevalence, frequency and/or quantity of alcohol consumed. According to the WHO, questions disaggregated by type of beverage consumed produce higher prevalence of consumption. The disadvantage is that questions disaggregated by type of beverage imply either that only one type of beverage is indicated or that if the option is taken to disaggregate the set of questions for each type of beverage, the questionnaire becomes too long and repetitive for respondents. Many of the studies inquire about four different types of beverages, namely wine, beer, alcopops (fruity drinks with low alcoholic content) and spirits/distilled beverages (whisky, brandy, etc.). This is the case in Portugal's National survey on drug use among general population, where frequency of consumption in the last year and frequency (in number of times and number of days) in the last month for each of these types of drink is asked. Portugal's first National Health Survey (1987) asked about the frequency in the last week of consumption of wine, beer, marc and brandy, and alcoholic beverages other than those mentioned. Besides the frequency of consumption of these types of beverages in the last week, it was also possible to know the quantities and number of occasions of consumption of wine and beer. In subsequent surveys, the frequency of consumption in the last week and the quantities and number of occasions of consumption of wine, beer, marc/brandy, port/vermouth/liqueurs and whisky/gin were also asked.

Another issue to be taken into account in indicators of consumption prevalence and patterns is the size of drinks. A large number of the questionnaires refer to standardised drinks, not specifying the size. There are two ways of presenting the amount of ethanol contained in a beverage. When collecting data on the type of beverage consumed, one can refer to the size/volume of the beverage (for example, the number of 330ml beers or 200ml glasses of wine, etc.) and multiply this information by the amount of ethanol contained in each amount of beverage, according to the reference table. The amount of ethanol in each drink, as mentioned above, differs from country to country. However, there are other factors that may influence the amount of ethanol to some extent: for example, in the case of wine, bottle sizes and the amount of ethanol vary greatly; distilled drinks are often mixed with other drinks or with ice, and this may be done by someone other than the respondent, who may not be aware of the amount of alcohol consumed.

The use of pictures of glasses or bottles is one of the alternatives to enable the respondent to indicate the kind of consumption in question. Portugal's national health surveys ask about the number of glasses and/or bottles and the volume of each one, as did the last two INPG applications and the RARHA.

One of the indicators of the circumstances and modes of consumption that we considered, and which is interrelated with the quantification of consumption by occasion, is drunkenness. The question of the frequency with which drunkenness occurs makes it possible to define the extent of one-off consumption, or on one occasion.

It should be borne in mind, however, that the state of drunkenness may be interpreted differently from culture to culture, and even within a single country this can vary over time, which can make comparison difficult. National surveys on consumption of substances in the general population in Portugal use this indicator.

The ages of onset and cessation of alcohol consumption are also surveyed in a large number of questionnaires. The reasons that lead an individual to consume also appear in a reasonable number of surveys, as well as the reasons for not consuming or quitting. The contexts of alcohol consumption is more rarely measured. Although these contexts are important to understand the association between consumption and the consequences associated with it, many studies do not take them into account. Generally, consumption contexts mean aspects such as where and with whom alcohol is consumed. According to the WHO, when using the last seven days as the reference period, it is important to associate the type of drink with the place and company of consumption. When the principle of generalised consumption is used, there are three questions to measure context, each of which may apply to the place where consumption occurs or to the company: 1) the respondent may be asked about the context in which consumption usually occurs or, alternatively, all the contexts in which consumption occurs; 2) respondents may also be asked to identify the proportion of time spent in different consumption contexts; 3) respondents may be asked about the frequency with which they drink in certain contexts.

Also, according to the WHO, the most usual ways of measuring high-risk consumption and the development of serious problems are the number or proportion of consumers and the total population whose consumption is problematic in a given period of time. The threshold of what is considered high-risk consumption is generally based on scientific criteria and may reflect national strategies based on a consumption pattern considered as moderate. In fact, the interest in measuring the level of abusive consumption in a country is precisely to prove the effectiveness of and adherence to prevention programmes. The most usual way to check exposure to a high risk of consumption is to ask whether the individual consumes six or more drinks per day/occasion (in the case of men) or four or more drinks per day/occasion (women) — or binge drinking. The amount of ethanol assumed depends on the country in question and has different patterns depending on whether consumption is by men or women. The measurement of high risk using the prevalence of consumption in the past seven days is not recommended to estimate the proportion of the population who drink to excess (generally, estimated consumption of 60 g of ethanol per day); this is because the proportion of individuals with this pattern of consumption is in most cases underestimated. Again, the context and the objectives of the survey have a lot of influence on the indicators of problematic consumption used. National health surveys tend to measure problematic or high-risk consumption mostly by the volume of alcohol ingested, whereas problematic or high-risk consumption in questionnaires on psychoactive substance tend to be measured not only by the quantity of alcohol ingested, but also by purpose-built tests such as the DSM-IV (Kandel et al. 1997), the Ontario Alcohol and Other Drug Opinion Survey (Ferris et al. 1994), the ALAC — Alcohol Advisory Council of New Zealand (ALAC 1996) or the AUDIT — Alcohol Use Disorders Identification Test (Saunders et al. 1993), among others. The biggest difficulty where the indicator of problematic consumption of alcohol is concerned seems to be the various concepts associated with it—dependence, abusive consumption, harmful consumption, problematic consumption, among others—with each of these presenting subtle distinctions, in medical and/or social terms.

Problems inherent to use of data on per capita alcohol consumption

According to the World Health Organization (WHO 2000), estimates of per capita alcohol consumption should be used with caution, as they can present three problems: what they do not measure, what they cannot measure, and the reliability or unreliability of the data on which they are based. These problems and suggested strategies for dealing with them are summarised in the following table and discussed below.

Table 7-3. Factors impairing the accuracy of per capita alcohol consumption estimates

Factor	Impact	Corrections
Informal production	Omission can lead to the underestimation of adult per capita alcohol consumption	Use periodic local surveys to estimate extent of local consumption of informally produced alcohol, and add this to the numerator of the adult per capita consumption formula
Tourist consumption	Omission can lead to overstating native consumption, underestimating consumption in tourists' home countries	a) correct adult per capita consumption formula in denominator to include estimate of annual tourist population; or b) correct adult per capita consumption formula in numerator by estimating tourist consumption (via special tax or marking on beverages slated for tourists) and subtracting it
Overseas consumption	Omission can lead to underestimation of national consumption	Derive estimate through inclusion of questions regarding quantity and frequency of overseas consumption in national surveys, and add this to the numerator of the adult per capita consumption formula
Stockpiling	Can cause national consumption to appear negative, as exports for a given year may exceed the sum of domestic production and imports	Correct adult per capita consumption formula in numerator by adding the difference between additional stocks available at the start of the year and those remaining at the end of the year.
Waste and spillage	Can cause an overestimate of national consumption	Include questions in periodic surveys to gain estimates of amounts of these
Smuggling	Omission can lead to underestimation of national consumption	Obtain estimate from law enforcement and tax collection officials of amount of alcohol smuggled into the country, and add to numerator of adult per capita consumption formula

Duty-free sales	Omission can lead to underestimation of national consumption	Derive estimates through inclusion of question regarding quantity and frequency of duty-free purchasing in national surveys, and add to numerator of adult per capita consumption formula
Variation in beverage strength	Can lead to inaccurate estimation of amount of pure alcohol consumed	Use domestic market share data to estimate median alcohol strength for each beverage category and significant subcategory

Source: Table from *International Guide for Monitoring Alcohol Consumption and Harm*, 2000, 29.

Estimates of per capita alcohol consumption are generally derived from data on the sale, production, trade and taxation of alcoholic beverages. As such, they rarely include measurements of informal production and consumption. Data are also lacking on the amount of consumption of duty-free (in some countries, for example Spain and Portugal, wine is exempt from excise duty) or contraband alcohol, as well as the amount of alcohol that residents consume abroad.

National surveys can play an important role in filling such gaps by including questions on the extent of duty-free purchases (that is, alcohol purchased for consumption in the country, in shops abroad or in duty-free shops at domestic points of entry), as well as the amount and frequency of alcohol consumption while abroad.

Estimates of per capita alcohol consumption may also mask the impact of tourism. A correction in these cases is possible if consumption data for natives and for tourists are available. Such data sources can be developed using separate markings, licensing or taxes for beverages sold to tourists. If such data do not exist and data on the size of tourism are available, a rough correction can be made by estimating the total annual population of tourists (for example, dividing by 365 the total number of days that tourists aged over 14 spent in the country) and adding the value obtained to the denominator in the formula for per capita alcohol consumption.

Finally, per capita measurements also do not provide insight into the impact of storage within the country, as is common in the production of beverages that require ageing, such as whiskey or brandy. Large producers of these beverages may have years in which exports exceed the sum of production and imports, because a large part of the batch produced in the previous year reached maturity and was used for export.

If estimates can be obtained of the extent of consumption of tax-free alcohol and alcohol produced at home or informally, consumption abroad, consumption by tourists, the volume of alcohol imported and re-exported to other countries, and the quantity of stored goods that enter the market — the ideal formula for estimating per capita alcohol consumption would be as follows:

$$\frac{\text{(alcohol production + alcohol imports + informal alcohol production + consumption overseas + duty-free consumption – tourist consumption – alcohol exports – alcohol re-exports + additional stocks)}}{\text{Population aged 15 or over}}$$

This is difficult to determine accurately.

Estimates of per capita alcohol consumption can measure only limited variations in a population. Consumption patterns within nations or cultures are extremely important. The more knowledge that can be gained about consumption patterns, as well as per capita consumption, the more accurately policies can be designed to reduce alcohol-related problems.

It is important to know rates of abstinence from alcohol consumption when seeking to make international comparisons using per capita consumption data.

Sales data can sometimes be useful in identifying patterns of consumption in terms of the use of different beverages, some of which may be of greater concern than others — for example, beers with low versus medium alcohol content (generally the cheaper varieties of beer are preferred by high-risk drinkers and their sales may be a marker of high-risk drinking). When making international comparisons using per capita alcohol consumption data, it is important to remember that countries have different socioeconomic and demographic profiles.

Levels and patterns of alcohol consumption also vary across countries according to the age of the consumer. Older people tend to drink less, and younger people tend to drink more, both overall and per day of consumption. Adjusting estimates of per capita alcohol consumption for age is recommended for some purposes, in order to assess whether observed changes or differences in total per capita consumption are due to underlying disparities in the age distributions of the populations studied. To make such age-standardised comparisons, it is necessary to have representative national survey data using comparable methodologies that allow estimates of typical drinking volumes for each age group, and for men and women.

Other aspects of drinking patterns are best assessed through population surveys and fieldwork of an ethnographic nature.

Finally, the data used for estimates of per capita alcohol consumption can come from many sources and be collected through a variety of methods. Their reliability may be difficult to assess, and measures may not be strictly comparable across countries. According to the Portuguese Observatory of Health Systems (OPSS), regarding WDT — World Drink Trends 2003 data listing the world's eight largest consumers at the time, Portugal was the only country with unreliable statistical data on alcohol consumption (OPSS 2003, 32).

The formula for estimating per capita alcohol consumption requires production and trade figures to be converted into litres of pure alcohol, which requires estimates or assumptions about the alcohol content of various beverages. Periodic national efforts should thus be made to estimate the median alcohol content of each beverage category, as values can vary widely from country to country.

In the absence of measurements at national level, the central question remains: what estimates should be used? Obtaining an international standard does not seem possible, due to the wide variation in alcohol content of the three beverage categories (beer, wine and spirits) from country to country (for example, the alcohol content of beer can vary from 0.5% to 14%). It should also be borne in mind that the three categories do not capture all alcoholic beverages consumed worldwide, nor the variation in alcohol content that can occur within a category. In this context, international consensus on the alcohol content of the various categories may in fact not be desirable and is a poor second option for transparent and well-founded estimates of alcohol content made at the national level.

In summary, let us now look at how per capita alcohol consumption can be estimated.

Per capita consumption figures should be calculated for the main categories of alcoholic beverages available in a country. Most international sources limit these categories to beer, distilled spirits and wine and consider them as a minimum reference; other categories should be added for local beverages that represent a substantial proportion of local consumption and that have an alcohol content that does not easily break down into one of the three main categories.

The following formula has been commonly used to estimate per capita alcohol consumption (Smart 1991 apud WHO 2000):

$$\frac{\text{Alcohol production} + \text{alcohol imports} - \text{alcohol exports}}{\text{Population aged 15 or over}}$$

Currently WHO estimates of per capita alcohol consumption take into account recorded and unrecorded alcohol and tourist consumption.

The measurement of adult per capita consumption is preferable to simple per capita consumption, due to the varying age structure of national populations. Per capita consumption figures based on total population tend to underestimate consumption in countries with larger proportions of the population under 15 years of age.

A more realistic approximation of actual consumption patterns can be obtained using the following formula, which combines estimates of adult per capita consumption with prevalence estimates drawn from representative national surveys, if accessible.

$$\frac{\text{Annual per capita alcohol consumption}}{\text{\% of consuming population aged 15 or over}} \times \frac{100}{365}$$

In general population surveys it is possible, from the existing information for each type of alcoholic beverage, to construct an annual estimate of alcohol consumption. The frequency of consumption of a specific quantity of an alcoholic beverage is used to provide further information on the usual patterns of consumption based on the annual frequency and habitual amount of consumption of beer, wine and spirits. This estimate allows the annual consumption of each individual alcoholic beverage to be calculated, as well as the total annual consumption of alcohol.

This estimate of annual consumption may not be sufficient to calculate comparable and accurate consumption levels. As has been confirmed over half a century of research by members of the RARHA team responsible for this topic, surveys fail to capture all alcohol consumption as recorded by sales statistics. In fact, the opposite is true: in the vast majority of research the so-called coverage rate can vary between 30% and 60% of the figure obtained from sales statistics (Moskalewicz, Room and Thom 2016).

In contrast, measuring alcohol consumption from national surveys allows information that cannot be gathered from routine statistics, as mentioned before. Firstly, these surveys make it possible to collect data on the proportion of the population that consumes alcoholic beverages and how this consumption is distributed across different sociodemographic groups, such as by gender and age. The collection of information through general population surveys also provides data on the frequency of alcohol consumption, the volume of consumption per occasion and the prevalence of high-risk consumption — crucial data for the formulation, implementation and evaluation of public policies to prevent alcohol consumption (Alanko 1984; Mäkelä 2006).

However, the World Health Organization, in its *International Guide for Monitoring Alcohol Consumption and Harm*, does not recommend the use of national survey data as a basis for calculating estimates of per capita alcohol consumption. According to the WHO, despite the importance of general population survey results for public policy purposes, in terms of who is consuming, how, how much and how often, these results show substantial discrepancies with per capita consumption estimates based on sales statistics (WHO 2000, 28). Nevertheless, it seems to us that some of these discrepancies may be related to flaws in the estimates based on sales data and, as mentioned above, in their translation into per capita consumption.

CHAPTER 8

RESULTS OF MEASUREMENT OF CONSUMPTION OF ALCOHOLIC BEVERAGES

Sources of statistical information

Global sources

The largest statistical sets relating to alcohol production and trade are those of the Food and Agriculture Organization (FAO) and the United Nations Statistical Office. The former publishes the most comprehensive sets of statistics available on the production of and trade in beer, wine and spirits, providing data on their production, exports and imports since 1961.

These statistics are available on the FAO website, which allows limited downloading of its data. However, the consistency of these data relies on the accuracy of the information provided by member states and the FAO's own ability, in the absence of reports from the countries themselves, to estimate production and trade. These data underestimate the amount of informal and domestic production of alcoholic beverages. They are sometimes incomplete, unavailable or presented as estimates for several years in a row. Data for most developed countries are made available by states themselves, by the alcohol industry or by organisations such as the commodity board of the distilling industry. These data are published by *World Drink Trends* (Productschap voor Gedistilleerde Dranken 1997), which uses almost 100 sources to estimate trends in alcohol consumption in 35 developed and 21 developing countries.

When production and trade statistics are used, we have to bear in mind the following precautions: 1) the figures generally quantify only formal—that is, large-scale industrial—alcohol production and trade, as opposed to informal, low-tech or domestic production and trade; 2) sometimes the FAO fills in gaps by estimating the data — a method that usually translates into repeating the production figures reported in the previous year. With population growth in many countries, this estimation method may point to per capita consumption reducing even when this is not the case. Gaps in the data can lead to false impressions of trends.

As seen above, estimates of adult per capita consumption of alcohol may provide evidence of long-term trends, but say little about actual consumption in the population. In countries where most consumption is by a minority—for example, men from a single ethnic or religious group—per capita figures can mask the extent of alcohol consumption. A clear picture of who drinks, how often, how much they drink, and with whom, can be constructed through data collected in population-based drinking surveys (which, as we have seen, have limitations at other levels).

If available, country-level data are preferable to those drawn from international sources. Also, sales data are generally preferable to production and trade data for estimating per capita consumption, provided that they are clearly differentiated from sales of other goods in retailers that sell alcohol. Government statistical offices and customs departments usually keep careful records of alcoholic beverages volumes and revenues for the purpose of monitoring taxes and duties. These figures can also be used to estimate adult per capita consumption. Taxes collected at producer level may introduce a lag in the data as they do not reflect actual retail sales. Sales data provided by the industry itself can also be used, where available.

In the absence of tax data, the production and trade data that often exist at the national level may be used, although they do not appear in the global sources.

Portuguese Food Balance Sheet

The Portuguese Food Balance Sheet (BAP) is a statistical analytical tool that makes it possible to portray the availability of foods in Portugal and, so far as we are concerned, those of alcoholic beverages. The BAP tracks the evolution of this availability, in terms of products, nutrients and calories, but does not characterise the consumption of the country's residents. However, as the 2013 report states, "given that the correlation coefficients between the BAP (food availabilities) and the Household Budget Survey — IDEF (quantities purchased by resident households), showed positive, high and statistically significant correlations in the common reference periods

(2005 and 2010), food availabilities are an indirect way of characterising food consumption" (INE 2014, 2) and, therefore, the consumption of alcoholic beverages.

Food consumption is measured from a food supply perspective, being "expressed as daily edible availabilities per inhabitant, translated into calories, protein, carbohydrates, fat and alcohol." (INE 2017, 3) The BAP food availability data include existing the quantities of beverages for consumption by residents of Portugal, both inside households and outside (in restaurants, canteens, hospitals, prisons, etc.) (INE 2014, 23).

Sources in the alcoholic beverage industry

Alcohol industry associations and market research firms use various methodologies to estimate global trends in the production, trade and consumption of alcoholic beverages. *World Drink Trends* (1997), compiled by the Dutch Distillers Association, draws on almost 100 published and unpublished sources, including United Nations and FAO statistics, but also figures requested directly from ministries and statistical institutes in particular countries and from alcohol industry associations. *World Drink Trends* attempts to estimate consumption in over 50 countries from all sources – domestic production, illicit production, consumption by tourists, duty-free sales, cross-border alcohol traffic and contraband.

For Portugal, statistical data on consumption of beer since 1954, wine since 1955, and spirits since 1964 are available. However, as mentioned above, these statistics are unsatisfactory since they do not cover all wine production, such as small-scale production for domestic use.

Instituto da Vinha e do Vinho, I.P.

At national level we can also refer to the Instituto da Vinha e do Vinho (IVV — Institute of Vine and Wine), a public institute that forms part of the state's indirect administration, with administrative and financial autonomy. Within the scope of its competences, it collects and provides statistical data on the sector.

The IVV website contains data on the reality of Portugal's wine sector, namely some information covering wine production in Portugal and its distribution across the wine-growing regions, by type of wine, production structure and scale of production, as well as data on consumption, imports and exports of wine. The data on wine consumption available on the site comes from the International Organisation of Vine and Wine — OIV.

Public health compendia and databases

Various research studies have drawn upon the above sources to summarize world trends in alcohol consumption from a public health perspective. In 1985, the WHO published a summary of world alcohol production trends, based solely on UN production data (Walsh and Grant 1985). In 1994, the Addiction Research Foundation published *International profile: alcohol and other drugs*, in collaboration with the World Health Organization (WHO 1994). Although it included tables on alcohol consumption, there was little new information, as the data presented originated from *World Drink Trends* and the two UN sources mentioned above. The WHO Regional Office for Europe produced a set of profiles of alcohol consumption and associated problems in the 1990s, targeting European countries with the aim of helping monitoring progress in achieving the European Alcohol Action Plan (Harkin 1995). Using country-level informants, as well as production and trade data from the UN and *World Drink Trends*, the profiles included estimates of per capita consumption of recorded alcohol, as well as information on unrecorded production where accessible.

The World Health Organization (2000) drew on work from Europe and other regions to publish the first *Global Status Report on Alcohol* (1999), followed by others in 2004, 2011, 2014 and 2018. These include estimates of adult per capita consumption in most countries, drawing on a combination of national and regional estimates, industry data and data from the FAO and the UN Statistical Office.

The WHO began collecting data in 1996 with the Global Alcohol Database, which was subsequently developed into the Global Information System on Alcohol and Health (GISAH[58]), starting in 2008. The GISAH serves as a repository of all key indicators presented in the country profiles, relying on global information on alcohol consumption and alcohol-related problems as well as considering related policy responses, and is organised

[58] http://www.who.int/globalatlas/alcohol

according to several categories, namely the "consumption levels" category, which includes major indicators of total per capita alcohol consumption, recorded consumption (in time series going back to 1960), consumption of unrecorded alcohol and tourist consumption; the "drinking patterns" category refers to indicators such as the prevalence of abstinence and episodic excessive consumers (World Health Organization 2018).

Thus, the Global Information System on Alcohol and Health (GISAH) serves to collect, compile, analyse and disseminate global information on alcohol and health. Within GISAH, data are organised under a broad set of seven categories: levels of alcohol consumption; consumption patterns; harms and consequences; economic aspects; alcohol control policies; prevention, research and treatment; and youth and alcohol. It currently covers over 150 indicators (many of them comparable across countries) related to alcohol, and has data from over 225 countries and territories.

National population-based studies

Portugal consistently ranks amongst the highest consumers of alcohol and alcoholic drinks in Europe and worldwide when we look at statistics from commerce and industry. However, in 2001 Portugal, along with Greece, Ireland, France and Belgium, was among the European countries with the fewest specialised studies undertaken specifically on alcohol consumption and its associated problems (Simpura et al. 2001). Today, 20 years later, the number of sources of population-based data and information about alcohol consumption in our country has increased substantially (INSA 2001; Gameiro 2000; Balsa et al. 2003, 2008, 2011, 2014, 2018; INE/INSA 2009, 2016; IAN-AF 2015/16).

In this report we shall focus on the national survey on drug use among general population (INPG)—mainly using data from the last application (2016/2017), but also presenting a longitudinal perspective (between 2001 and 2017)—as well as on Reducing Alcohol Related Harm (RARHA, Portugal 2015).

The Reducing Alcohol Related Harm (RARHA) joint action, already mentioned above, had as its main objective, in *Workpackage 4 — Monitoring, Task 1* (named RARHA SEAS — *Reducing Alcohol Related Harm — Standardised European Alcohol Survey*), to use the SMART

(Standardizing Measurement of Alcohol Related Troubles) questionnaire as a model for the collection of comparable data on drinking patterns and their harmful effects in the European Union Member States.

The fourth national survey on drug use among general population (INPG), Portugal 2016/17 was promoted by SICAD (the General Directorate for Intervention on Addictive Behaviours and Dependencies), and conducted by CICS.NOVA — Interdisciplinary Centre of Social Sciences, and follows those conducted in 2001, 2007 and 2012, making it possible to consolidate knowledge on the evolution of the prevalence of use of licit and illicit substances. The information collected allows the creation of consumer profiles, as well as an evaluation of the perception of risk that the population has towards certain behaviours and the perception of availability of substances, prevalence and problems associated with gambling and internet use, among others (see the more detailed presentation in the next section).

In both studies, the universe is the population living in mainland Portugal and in the Autonomous Regions of Azores and Madeira, aged between 15 and 74 (in both cases, inclusive) in the case of the INPG, and between 18 and 64 (in both cases, inclusive) for RARHA. Only the population living in family homes is included, leaving out the population living in institutions (barracks, convents, prisons, residences for students or the elderly, etc.), the population living in collective establishments (hotels, boarding houses, etc.) and the homeless population.

The sample design followed in both studies is probabilistic and representative of the populations targeted (as will also be presented below).

The sample size is, in the case of RARHA, 1,500 respondents and, in the case of INPG, 9,632 individuals for the population aged between 15 and 64 and 12,023 when considering the population aged 15 to 74.

In both studies the fieldwork was carried out by the company Intercampus S.A. in strict compliance with the rules of conduct of the ICC/Esomar Code and Portugal's Data Protection Law no. 67/98 of 26 October.

Information collection took place, in the case of RARHA, between June and September 2015 and, in the case of INPG, between December 2016 and June 2017, with a control collection taking place in September 2017.

In both RARHA and INPG, computer-assisted personal interviewing (CAPI) was applied.

The response rate to the RARHA questionnaire was 61% and that for the INPG was 57.1%.

In both studies, the results are weighted in order to correct distortions suffered by the sample when we decided not to fully respect the proportionality of the population weight in the regions, with the aim of ensuring a comfortable sample in the less populated regions, thus lowering the margins of sampling error. The correction of the sample is also justified by the small distortions that may occur during the sample planning and collection operations. The sampling errors arise from the fact that the questionnaires were distributed to the regions taking into account a breakdown of the estimated population.

The methodology of Jacinto Rodríguez Osuna (1991, 1993) was followed to calculate the error margins. This technique corrects the error calculation formula for a random sample, with the results of the calculations of the effect of the sample design adopted (multistage sampling stratified by clusters). The calculations were made for a confidence level of 95%, and the minimum and maximum intervals are presented in the tables regarding prevalence.

Measuring consumption: indicators and results

The diversity of strategies followed to measure consumption, as is clear from the descriptions we have presented, certainly reflects the complexity of the objective. The ways of responding to resolve consumption-related problems are made denser at three levels: 1) on the one hand, there are national political cultures, organisational cultures or even the cultures of the research devices themselves; 2) on the other hand, these idiosyncrasies are themselves strongly rooted in local cultures, which can themselves change; 3) finally, consumption patterns at national level are not equally distributed among the respective populations and may have very diverse consequences.

Regardless of how this diversity affects the definition of the social or cultural frameworks of the problems, we are interested in understanding how it can condition the measures of two crucial variables from the health perspective: the amount of alcohol consumed and frequency of consumption. To this end, we will review the sources we presented earlier.

Global, national and industry statistics and public health bases

Alcohol consumption levels can be measured using various indicators, with two of the most important and most commonly used being total alcohol consumption per capita/year in litres of pure alcohol and alcohol consumption in grams of pure alcohol per person/day. The recorded per capita alcohol consumption is part of a basic set of indicators, whose purpose is to monitor the magnitude, pattern and trends of alcohol consumption in the adult population.

The World Health Organization, through the Global Information System on Alcohol and Health (GISAH), provides data from 1961 on per capita alcohol consumption, namely for the European Region, including Portugal.

GISAH defines per capita *recorded* alcohol consumption as the amount of alcohol consumed by adults (aged 15+) over the course of a calendar year in a country, in litres of pure alcohol. The indicator takes into account only consumption that is recorded in production, import, export and sales data, often known through tax collection.

The per capita alcohol consumption indicator is based on estimates of consumption of recorded and unrecorded alcohol; the latter represents alcohol that is not taxed and is outside the usual system of government control because it is produced, distributed and sold outside formal channels and therefore not recorded by routine data collection (Rehm et al. 2003, 2007). It is essential to include unrecorded consumption in estimates of overall levels of alcohol exposure in populations, because more than a quarter of global alcohol consumption can be attributed to it (WHO 2011).

Many national governments regularly monitor per capita alcohol consumption and make reliable data available. It is these statistics that garner the highest preference in reports in the GISAH, when they are validated. However, even if national statistics are not available, per capita consumption can be estimated either through public data provided by industry or using data provided by the FAO statistical database (FAOSTAT). An algorithm is used by the WHO Secretariat to validate the data[59] and decide which statistics to opt for.

Obviously, unrecorded consumption is more difficult to estimate and monitor, and only a few countries do so. For all others, unrecorded alcohol

---

[59] For more information, see http://who.int/gho/gisah.

consumption is estimated from studies and expert opinion. In the 2012 *Global Survey on Alcohol and Health* a module developed and implemented based on the principles of the Delphi survey methodology on unrecorded alcohol consumption (Linstone and Turoff 1975, Rehm and Gadenne 1990) was added to the main questionnaire.

This module covers estimates of unrecorded alcohol consumption in its main categories: home production (of spirits, wine and beer), cross-border alcohol (smuggling, duty-free and cross-border purchases), illegal production (including counterfeit alcoholic beverages) and alcohol substitutes (liquids generally containing ethanol and industrial alcohol not intended for consumption as a beverage). The questionnaire also addresses the representation of the importance of unrecorded alcohol consumption from a public health perspective, as well as the measures implemented at the national level to reduce the public health impact of illegal and informally produced alcohol, according to a set of policy options and interventions listed in the WHO's Global strategy to reduce the harmful use of alcohol (WHO 2010).

Tourist consumption is also considered in estimating alcohol consumption per capita in populations where it is significant (where the number of tourists per year is at least equal to the number of inhabitants) and is not balanced by the consumption of domestic inhabitants abroad during holidays.

Alcohol consumption per capita is an example of the indicators monitored via GISAH at national, regional and global levels. According to the World Health Organization database, Portugal had the following values for alcohol consumption per capita recorded for the population aged 15 or older between 1961 and 2018:

Table 8-1. Per capita consumption of recorded alcohol 1961-2018 (in litres of pure alcohol)

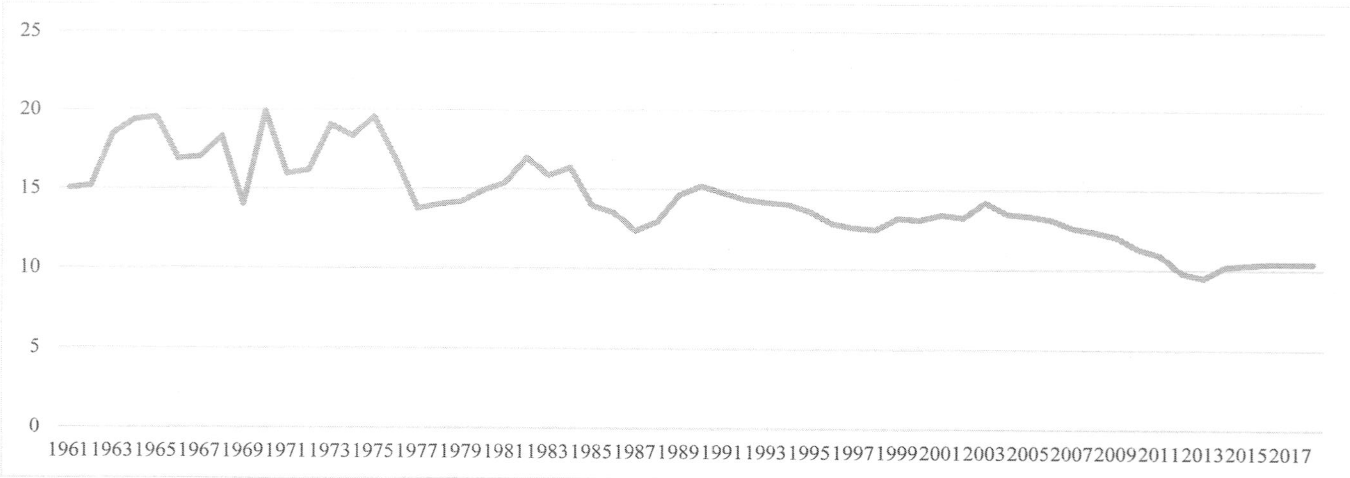

Source: Global Information System on Alcohol and Health (GISAH), World Health Organization (WHO).

After standing at around 20 litres of pure alcohol per year in the 1960s and 1970s, and 15 litres in the 1980s and 1990s, values have been declining since 2003, with estimates for 2016 being 10.4 litres of pure alcohol per year. The estimated per capita recorded alcohol consumption for 2016 and 2017 is 10.4 litres, representing a decrease from the 2010 estimate and following the trend of the WHO European Region as a whole.

Table 8-2. Per capita consumption of recorded alcohol 2001, 2007, 2012 and 2017, Portugal * (in litres of pure alcohol)

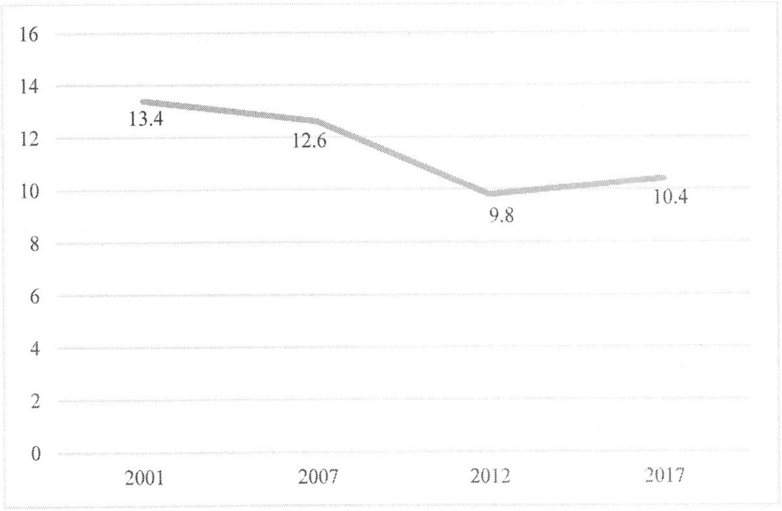

* Years when the survey was applied to the general population in Portugal (Balsa et al. 2003, 2009, 2014 & 2018).

Source: Global Information System on Alcohol and Health (GISAH), World Health Organization (WHO).

The World Health Organization calculates and makes available data on total alcohol consumption per capita in the Global Information System on Alcohol and Health (GISAH). This consumption is defined as the total amount (recorded + unrecorded) of alcohol consumed by adults (aged 15+) during a calendar year, in litres of pure alcohol, adjusted for tourist consumption.

The estimate of total alcohol consumption per capita is obtained by adding the three-year average of recorded alcohol consumption and the three-year average of unrecorded alcohol consumption, from which is subtracted the three-year average of tourist consumption, in a given calendar year. Tourist consumption considers tourists visiting the country and residents visiting other countries. Data are available by gender.

Table 8-3. Total per capita consumption of alcohol (recorded and unrecorded) 2000-2018, Portugal

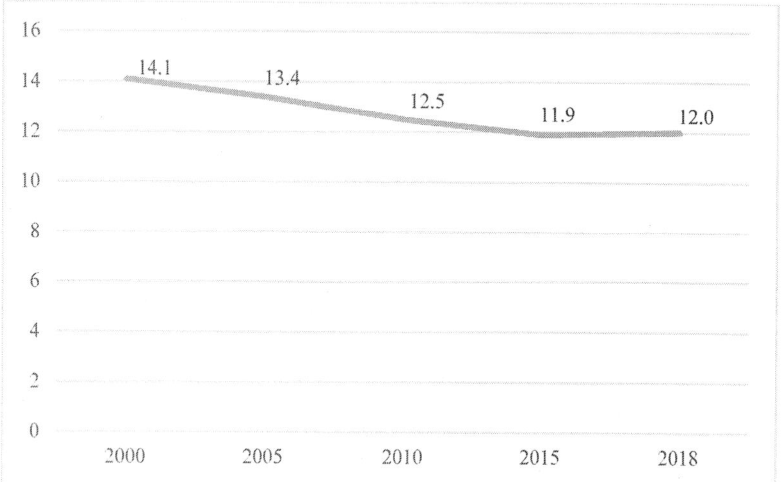

Source: Global Information System on Alcohol and Health (GISAH), World Health Organization (WHO). Last update on 8 April 2020.

Another important indicator to measure alcohol consumption is the prevalence of consumers and of abstainers. According to data from the Global Status Report on Alcohol and Health 2018, the number of lifetime abstainers in Portugal in 2016 is 12.6%, with a higher figure for women (18.4%) than for men (6.0%).

Table 8-4. Abstainers 2016 (%)

	Total	Men	Women
Lifetime abstainers*	12.6	6.0	18.4
Former drinkers**	18.2	12.4	23.3
Abstainers in last 12 months***	30.8	18.4	41.7

* People who have never consumed alcohol.

** People who have consumed alcohol, but have not done so in the last 12 months.

*** People who have not consumed alcohol in the last 12 months (lifetime abstainers + former drinkers).

Source: World Health Organization, 2018.

Table 8-5. Alcohol per capita (ages 15+) consumption (in litres of pure alcohol)

	Average 2003-2005	Average 2008-2010	Average 2009-2011	Average 2015-2017
Recorded alcohol	12.3	11.0	12.1	10.6
Unrecorded alcohol	2.1	1.9	1.9	2.1
Total*	14.4	12.9	13.5	12.3 (11.9-12.7)**
Total men	--	18.7	21.9	20.5 (19.8-21.2)**
Total women	--	7.6	5.9	5.1 (4.9-5.3)**
WHO European Region	11.9	10.9	11.2	9.8

* Adjusted for tourist consumption.

** 95% confidence interval.

Source: World Health Organization, 2014, 2018.

Figure 8-1 Recorded alcohol per capita (ages 15+) consumption (in litres of pure alcohol) by type of beverage, 2016

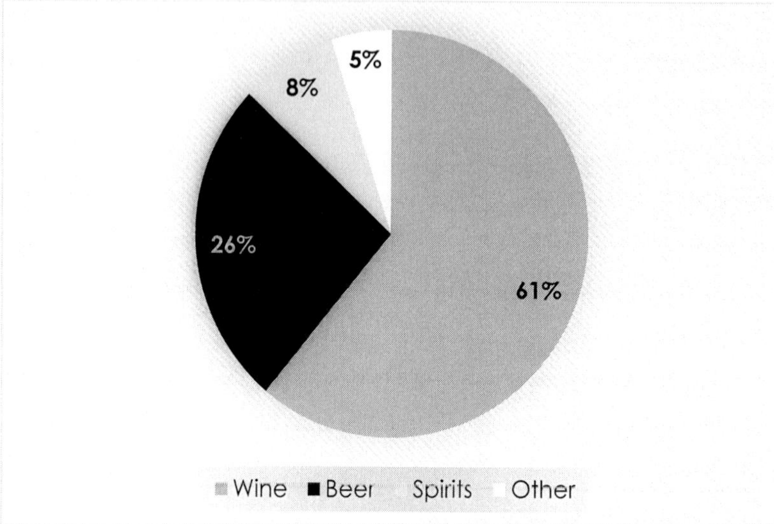

Source: World Health Organization, 2018.

Table 8-6. Prevalence of heavy episodic drinking* (%), 2016

	population (aged 15+)	drinkers only (aged 15+)	population (aged 15-19)	drinkers only (aged 15-19)
Total	26.6	38.4	29.9	51.5
Men	43.4	53.1	46.9	65.4
Women	11.9	20.3	12.8	28.9

* Consumption of 60 grams or more of pure alcohol on one occasion in the last 30 days.
Source: World Health Organization, 2018.

About a quarter (26.6%) of the population aged 15 or over say they have had an experience of binge drinking in the 30 days prior to the interview. If we limit the reference population only to alcohol users, this proportion naturally rises to 38.4%. These experiences are particularly significant for men (43.4% and 53.1% respectively).

Binge drinking is an experience that seems to be particularly significant among the youngest populations—15-19 years old—where occasional binge drinking rises to 29.9% or 51.5%, depending on whether we consider the entire population of the group or just alcohol users. In the case of men, the figures are 46.9% and 65.4% respectively.

These figures alert us to the difficulty of comparing results produced by different sources since, as mentioned above, both the reference populations and the measures are constructed on different assumptions. In the cases of occasional excessive consumption, for example, the table above considers the population living in Portugal aged 15 or over, which in 2017 represented 86% of the country's total population (at around 8,867,131 individuals)[60]. In the RARHA study, whose results we shall present below, as well as in the INPG, both of which we carried out, the reference population is aged between 15 and 64, which represents (for the same reference year) around 65% of the population.

We also know, from the most recent data obtained through the ECATD-CAD/2019 study, that 37% of respondents have consumed an alcoholic drink at the age of 13 or less and that, according to the same study, 21.1% of respondents aged 13 and 36.3% of those aged 14 had consumed alcohol in the last 12 months prior to the survey. This means that, as we mentioned at length in the first part, the way in which the target populations are constructed conditions the results obtained.

At another level, but still in order to underline the caution required when comparing results from different sources, we should bear in mind that the data used to measure per capita recorded alcohol consumption (for ages 15+) comes from *World Drink Trends* 1963-1999, as well as from GlobalData, from the OIV — Organisation Internationale de la Vigne et du Vin and from IWSR — International Wine and Spirits Research 2000-2016. As seen earlier, these data often rely, not on official national sources, but on industry estimates.

Portuguese Food Balance Sheet

The data presented by the Portuguese Food Balance Sheet coincides, on the whole, with that provided by the WHO (see above). Between 1990 and 2003 there was a change in the pattern of consumption, with alcoholic beverages

---

[60] Source: Resident population (No.) by Place of residence (NUTS — 2013), Sex and Age group; Annual — INE, Annual estimates of resident population.

losing relative importance, falling from 65% of the consumption structure to 42%, with the decrease in the importance of wine being pointed out as the main cause for this structural change: in fact, while daily per capita consumption of any beverage fell by 16% in this period, wine consumption fell by 25% (INE 2004, 5).

This evolution has, however, seen several oscillations during the period under review. Between 2003 and 2008 the amount available for daily per capita consumption of alcoholic beverages decreased by 8%. Beer emerges as the alcoholic beverage with the highest daily per capita availability (55% of the total in 2008), overtaking wine, whose availability decreased by around 10% (40% of total alcoholic beverages), continuing the trend that started in the 1990s (INE 2010, 11).

Between 2008 and 2012 this trend continued: the daily quantities of alcoholic beverages available per capita for consumption were 261.4ml/inhabitant/day, showing a decrease of 13.2%. The reduction was observed both for wine and beer—respectively 7.6 and 8.3 litres—with the latter remaining the alcoholic beverage with the highest quantity available for consumption (INE 2014, 16). All alcoholic beverages recorded a decrease in the quantities available. The increase in value-added tax (VAT) on alcoholic beverages is pointed out as a possible reason for these decreases (INE 2014, 17).

In 2016, the relative share of beer and wine in the daily available quantities per capita of alcoholic beverages remained the same: 50.5% and 44.8%, respectively, with the remaining quantity distributed among spirits, liqueurs and other distilled and fermented beverages.

Figure 8-2. Daily edible capitation of alcoholic beverages available for supply* (ml/inhabitant), 1990-2016

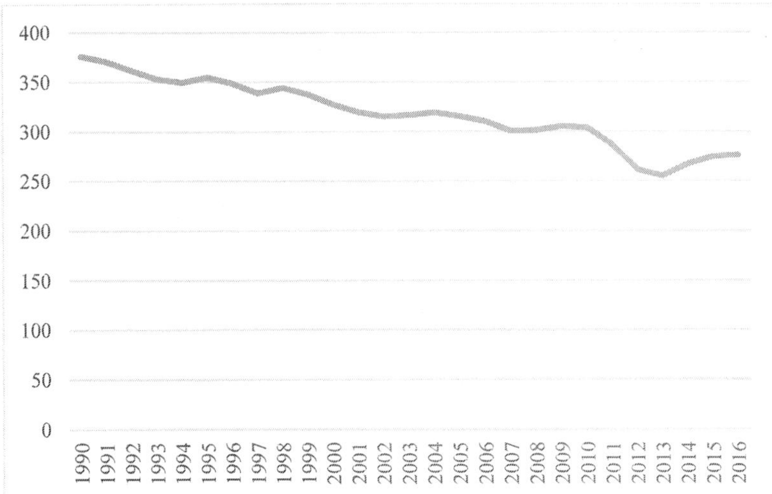

* Table of composition of foods 1999 for the years 1990 to 2011 and table of composition of foods 2016 for the years 2012 to 2016.

Source: Portuguese Food Balance Sheet, INE.

Figure 8-3. Daily capitation of alcohol available for supply (g/inhabitant), 1990-2016

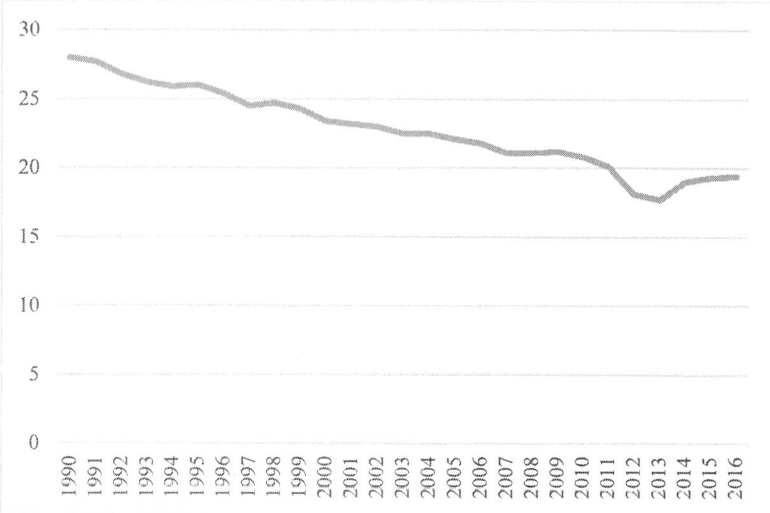

Source: Portuguese Food Balance Sheet, INE.

Table 8-7. Daily edible capitation of alcoholic beverages available for supply* (ml/inhabitant) by type of alcoholic beverage, 1990-2016

	1990	1991	1992	1993	1994	1995	1996	1997	1998	1999	2000	2001	2002
Total alcoholic beverages	376.1	370.7	361.7	353.2	349.7	354.8	348.6	338.7	344.2	337.6	327.3	319.5	315.3
Fermented alcoholic beverages	363	357.5	349.3	340.8	337.3	342.7	336.8	327.4	332.9	326.3	316.1	308	303.8
Wine and derivatives	173.4	172.1	166.3	162.5	159.7	157.5	153.2	147.1	145.5	139.5	131.2	131	129.9
Beer	185.8	181.6	179.2	174.2	174	181.4	179.2	175.9	181.9	180.8	178.9	171	167.9
Other fermented beverages	3.8	3.8	3.8	4.1	3.6	3.8	4.4	4.4	5.5	6	6	6	6
Other alcoholic beverages	13.1	13.2	12.4	12.4	12.4	12.1	11.8	11.3	11.3	11.3	11.2	11.5	11.5
Brandies (40% in alcohol by volume)	7.9	7.7	6.6	6.6	6.3	6.3	6	5.5	5.5	5.5	5.2	5.2	5.2
Liqueurs (25% in alcohol by volume)	1.4	1.4	1.4	1.4	1.4	1.1	1.1	1.1	1.1	1.1	1.1	1.1	1.1
Others (40% in alcohol by volume)	3.8	4.1	4.4	4.4	4.7	4.7	4.7	4.7	4.7	4.7	4.9	5.2	5.2

* Table of composition of foods 1999 for the years 1990 to 2011 and table of composition of foods 2016 for the years 2012 to 2016.

Table 8-7 continued.

	2003	2004	2005	2006	2007	2008	2009	2010	2011	2012	2013	2014	2015	2016
Total alcoholic beverages	316.5	319.2	315.4	310.2	300.6	301.2	305.2	303.8	286.5	261.1	255.1	266.8	274.4	276.1
Fermented alcoholic beverages	306.4	309.1	305.8	300.6	291	292.4	297.3	297	279.7	254.3	248.3	260.0	267.9	269.6
Wine and derivatives	130.7	129.9	128.8	126.6	120.5	124.4	130.7	130.7	129	109.0	105.8	121.9	123.8	123.8
Beer	169.9	173.4	171.5	168.8	164.7	162.2	160.8	160.5	145.2	139.5	136.2	131.8	137.8	139.5
Other fermented beverages	5.8	5.8	5.5	5.2	5.8	5.8	5.8	5.8	5.5	5.8	6.3	6.3	6.3	6.3
Other alcoholic beverages	10.1	10.1	9.6	9.6	9.6	8.8	7.9	6.8	6.8	6.8	6.8	6.8	6.5	6.5
Brandies (40% in alcohol by volume)	3.8	3.8	3.3	3.6	3.3	3.3	3	3	3	3.3	3.0	3.0	3.0	3.0
Liqueurs (25% in alcohol by volume)	1.1	1.1	1.1	1.1	1.4	1.1	1.1	1.1	1.1	0.8	1.1	0.8	0.8	0.8
Others (40% in alcohol by volume)	5.2	5.2	5.2	4.9	4.9	4.4	3.8	2.7	2.7	2.7	2.7	3.0	2.7	2.7

* Table of composition of foods 1999 for the years 1990 to 2011 and table of composition of foods 2016 for the years 2012 to 2016.
Source: Portuguese Food Balance Sheet, INE.

Table 8-8. Daily capitation of alcoholic beverages available for supply* (ml/inhabitant) by type of alcoholic beverage, 1990-2016

	1990	1991	1992	1993	1994	1995	1996	1997	1998	1999	2000	2001	2002
Total alcoholic beverages	28.0	27.7	26.8	26.2	25.9	26	25.4	24.5	24.7	24.3	23.4	23.2	23
Fermented alcoholic beverages	22.9	22.6	22	21.4	21.1	21.3	20.8	20.1	20.3	19.9	19	18.7	18.5
Wine and derivatives	15.6	15.5	15	14.6	14.4	14.2	13.8	13.2	13.1	12.6	11.8	11.8	11.7
Beer	6.9	6.7	6.6	6.4	6.4	6.7	6.6	6.5	6.7	6.7	6.6	6.3	6.2
Other fermented beverages	0.4	0.4	0.4	0.4	0.3	0.4	0.4	0.4	0.5	0.6	0.6	0.6	0.6
Other alcoholic beverages	5.1	5.1	4.8	4.8	4.8	4.7	4.6	4.4	4.4	4.4	4.4	4.5	4.5
Brandies (40% in alcohol by volume)	3.2	3.1	2.6	2.6	2.5	2.5	2.4	2.2	2.2	2.2	2.1	2.1	2.1
Liqueurs (25% in alcohol by volume)	0.4	0.4	0.4	0.4	0.4	0.3	0.3	0.3	0.3	0.3	0.3	0.3	0.3
Others (40% in alcohol by volume)	1.5	1.6	1.8	1.8	1.9	1.9	1.9	1.9	1.9	1.9	2	2.1	2.1

Table 8-8 continued.

	2003	2004	2005	2006	2007	2008	2009	2010	2011	2012	2013	2014	2015	2016
Total alcoholic beverages	22.5	22.5	22.1	21.8	21.1	21.1	21.2	20.8	20.1	18.1	17.7	19	19.3	19.4
Fermented alcoholic beverages	18.6	18.6	18.4	18.1	17.4	17.7	18.2	18.2	17.5	15.6	15.1	16.4	16.8	16.9
Wine and derivatives	11.8	11.7	11.6	11.4	10.8	11.2	11.8	11.8	11.6	9.9	9.6	11.1	11.3	11.3
Beer	6.3	6.4	6.3	6.2	6.1	6	5.9	5.9	5.4	5.2	4.8	4.6	4.8	4.9
Other fermented beverages	0.5	0.5	0.5	0.5	0.5	0.5	0.5	0.5	0.5	0.5	0.7	0.7	0.7	0.7
Other alcoholic beverages	3.9	3.9	3.7	3.7	3.7	3.4	3	2.6	2.6	2.5	2.6	2.6	2.5	2.5
Brandies (40% in alcohol by volume)	1.5	1.5	1.3	1.4	1.3	1.3	1.2	1.2	1.2	1.2	1.2	1.2	1.2	1.2
Liqueurs (25% in alcohol by volume)	0.3	0.3	0.3	0.3	0.4	0.3	0.3	0.3	0.3	0.2	0.3	0.2	0.2	0.2
Others (40% in alcohol by volume)	2.1	2.1	2.1	2	2	1.8	1.5	1.1	1.1	1.1	1.1	1.2	1.1	1.1

Source: Portuguese Food Balance Sheet, INE.

Instituto da Vinha e do Vinho, I.P.

In the particular case of wine, the structural downward trend in consumption or available quantities so far documented is not corroborated by the data provided for Portugal by the Instituto da Vinha e do Vinho (IVV — Institute of Vine and Wine) for the first 20 years of this century.

Figure 8-4. Evolution of wine consumption, 2000 to 2019 (million hl)

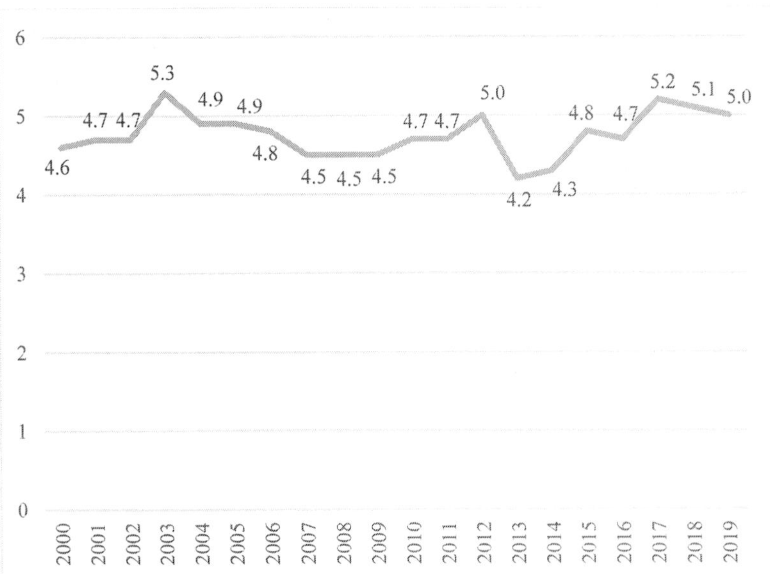

* Provisional data for 2018.

** Provisional data for 2019.

Source: Instituto da Vinha e do Vinho; OIV — Organisation Internationale de la Vigne et du Vin (The International Organisation of Vine and Wine).

Although the evolution is not linear, the curve points more towards a stabilisation of consumption levels, with decreases during the economic crises of 2007-2009 and the financial crisis of 2011-2013.

National population-based studies

As mentioned above, since this information comes from national population-based studies, we shall focus on the two surveys that we conducted in Portugal: the RARHA and the national survey on drug use among general population (INPG), applied since 2001.

The two studies have very different contexts of survey, questions and sample sizes. We shall, however, use the same age range: 15-64. To facilitate the reading of the figures, we shall put only the dates, with 2001, 2007, 2012 and 2017 referring to data from the I, II, III and IV INPG, and 2015 referring to data from RARHA.

Lifetime, last 12 months and last 30 days prevalence of alcohol consumption and abstinence

When we consider population-based studies, the downward trend in consumption pointed out by some of the sources presented above is also observed. The figure that follows details the distribution.

If we consider lifetime prevalence of alcohol consumption, we see that it steadily increases; from around 75% in 2001 it rises every year (with the exception of 2012, when it registers 73.6%) until it reaches 86.4% in 2017. This increase in lifetime consumption is probably justified by the maintenance of consumption cultures. The decrease in the 2012 application of the survey was explained in chapter 3 of the first part by a one-off change in the structure of the survey population, in addition to the margins of error in the results being higher than in other years. The collection carried out in 2015 re-establishes this continuity in what we can understand as an upward trend in consumption during the period under consideration.

We know, however, that the lifetime prevalence indicator is a measure that accumulates the consumption experiences of the population over time (a person who has consumed at some time continues to count towards the indicator, whatever their subsequent behaviour). If we consider, however, the updated record of consumption, we see that in fact the tendency is for prevalence to decrease.

Regarding last-year consumption, there is an increase between 2001 and 2007 from 65.9% to 70.6%, but a stabilisation in 2015 (70.9%) and a decrease in 2017 (59.4%).

As for current consumption, measured by the indicator for the last 30 days, this was around 60% in 2001 and 2007, and dropped to 49.1% in 2017, a reduction of almost 10 percentage points.

Figure 8-5. Prevalence of consumption of any alcoholic beverage (lifetime, last year and last month), 2001-2017 - population aged 15-64 (%)

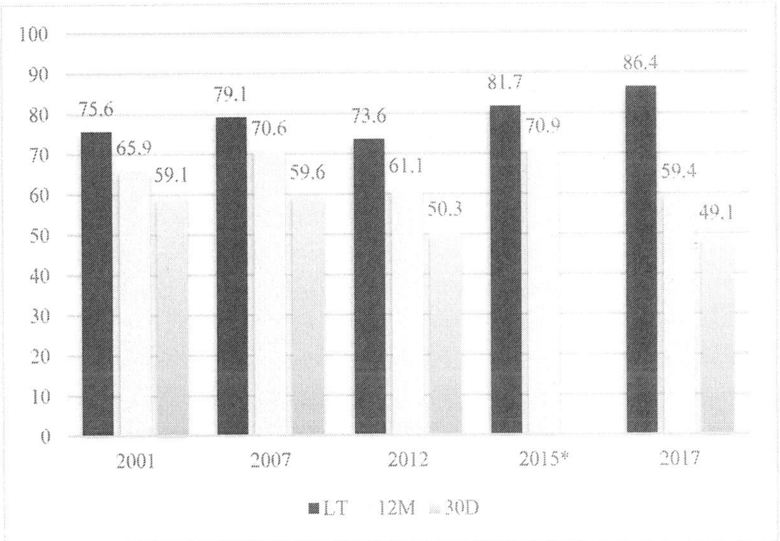

* There is no information for consumption in the last month in the RARHA study.
Source: I, II, III & IV INPG Portugal; RARHA 2015 for Portugal.

In all time periods, prevalence rates are higher in men than in women and also vary according to age: while over their lifetime young adults (aged 15-34) record lower prevalence rates than the population as a whole, the same is not true for the indicator of last-year consumption, which shows values quite similar to those of the total population in 2001, 2007 and 2012, but a somewhat sharp decline in 2017, for 51.6% in the young adult population and 59.4% in the total population. These results are detailed in the team's existing publications and will be put into perspective in a future publication.

Abstainers

Abstention is an important indicator in monitoring the health impact of global alcohol consumption and its assessment is critical to understanding epidemiological estimates (Rehm and Scafato 2011). There are two different types of abstainers — lifetime abstainers (those who have never consumed alcohol) and ex-drinkers/ex-consumers (people who have previously consumed alcohol but have not done so in the last 12 months). Together, these two subgroups constitute a group that can be described as last-year abstinent — people who have not consumed any alcoholic beverages in the last 12 months (WHO 2014). In epidemiological studies, alcohol abstinence is usually defined as a phenomenon related to current lifestyle (last year/last 12 months) rather than an immutable lifelong characteristic, because, as Rehm et al. (2008) showed, more than half of the respondents who in a survey defined themselves as lifetime abstinent had reported some alcohol consumption in previous surveys.

Abstainers (those who have not consumed alcohol in the last 12 months) are around 30% to 40% of the population between 2001 and 2017, reaching the highest percentage in the latter year, at 40.6%, a figure to which the increase in ex-consumers/people who have given up alcohol contributes a lot. The prevalence of last-year abstainers is higher among women.

Figure 8-6. Prevalence of abstainers. Data for Portugal 2001-2017

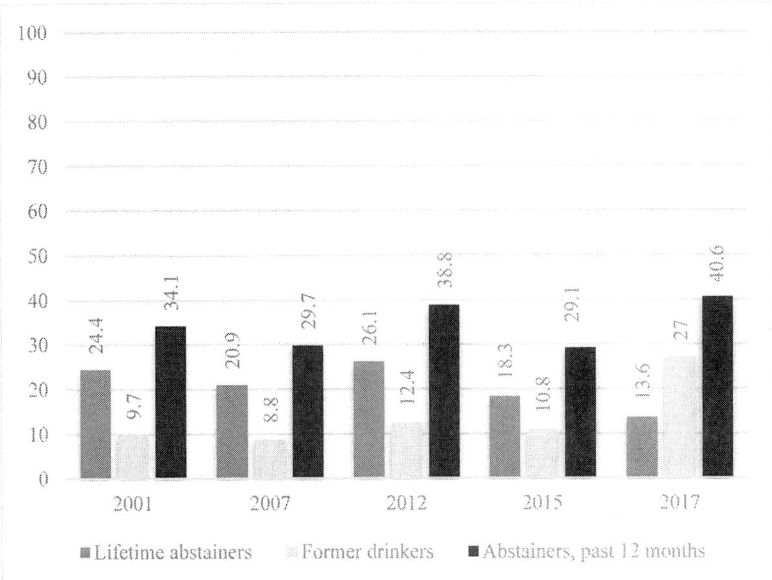

Source: I, II, III & IV INPG Portugal; RARHA 2015.

Frequency of consumption and types of beverages consumed (2015 and 2017)

Before analysing the actual frequency of consumption, it is important to reflect on the way the questions were asked in one or another questionnaire, what types of responses were chosen, and what filters exist, among other issues, in order to better understand the results.

In the RARHA study all respondents are asked: "Over the past 12 months, how often did you drink beer (not including light or alcohol-free)? Would you say you drank 'almost daily', 'weekly', 'monthly', 'less often' or 'never'?"; this question is also asked for wine, spirits and the frequency of any beverage. In a second step, these frequencies are detailed: "More specifically, would you say that in the last 12 months you drank ... — 1) Every day; 2) 5-6 days a week; 3) 3-4 days a week; 4) 1-2 days a week; 5) 2-3 days a month; 6) Once a month; 7) 6-11 days a year; 8) 2-5 days a year; 9) Once a year; 10) Did not drink beer in the last 12 months, but drank before; 11) Never drank beer, or just had a few sips."

From the frequency of consumption declared by the respondents, we can calculate, in addition to the frequencies, the prevalence of consumption, both lifetime and in the last 12 months.

In the 2017 INPG, meanwhile, the first two questions seek to gauge lifetime prevalence ("Have you ever, throughout your life, had any alcoholic drink, e.g. beer, wine or other beverage containing alcohol?") and in the last 12 months ("And during the last 12 months, have you had any alcoholic drink?"). The first question is put to all respondents, while the second question applies only to those who answered the first question in the affirmative. Thus, the question on frequency of consumption—"In the last 12 months, how often did you drink beer (not including light or alcohol-free)?" (repeated for each of the types of beverages considered)—is put only to those who consumed in the last 12 months.

The different way of asking the questions, the filters used in the questions, the different ways of answering, among others, influence the results and may affect the quality of the comparison.

According to the answers obtained through these questionnaires, of the three types of beverages considered, wine is the one with the highest prevalence rate, both in the 2015 study and in the 2017 study. Beer is the second most consumed type of beverage.

Figure 8-7. Type of beverage consumed 2015 and 2017 (population aged 15-64)

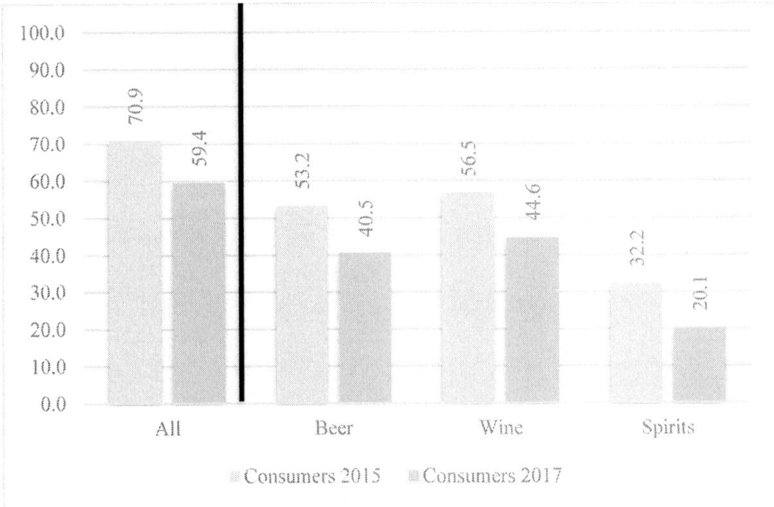

Source: RARHA 2015 and INPG 2017.

In addition to wine currently being the alcoholic beverage most consumed in Portugal, it is also the most regularly consumed: in 2015, it was consume once a week or more by 30.8%, with 14.7% consuming it daily; in 2017, wine was consumed once a week or more by 27.2%, with 13.9% consuming it daily; there is therefore a slight decrease in the most frequent consumption between the two applications. Also, beer drinkers, in both studies, show values of around 25% for consumption one or more times a week (25.8% in 2015 and 23.6% in 2017), although daily consumption for beer (at 5.4% in 2015 and 7.4% in 2017) is lower than that for wine. Spirits are mainly consumed fewer than six times a year.

Figure 8-8. Frequency of consumption in last 12 months by type of beverage I. RARHA 2015 and INPG 2017 (population aged 15-64) (%)

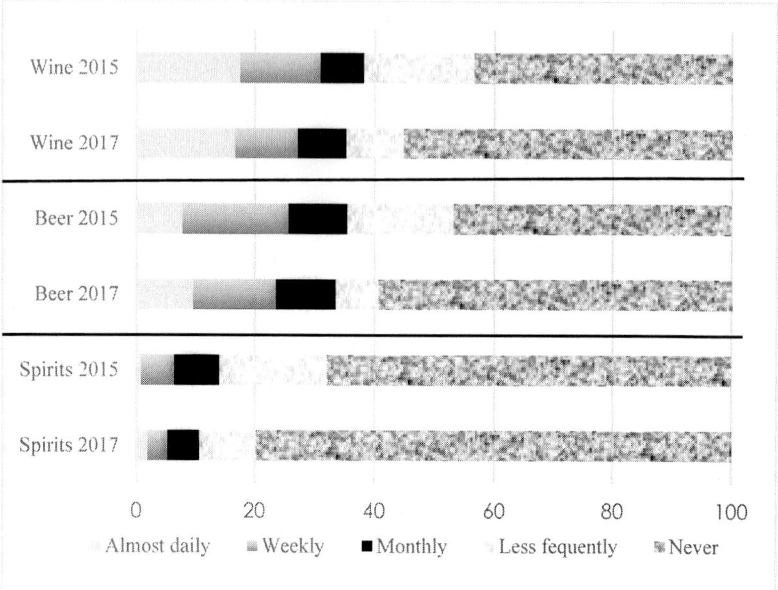

Source: RARHA 2015 and INPG 2017.

Table 8-9. Frequency of consumption in the last 12 months by type of beverage II. RARHA 2015 and INPG 2017 (population aged 15-64) (%)

	WINE		BEER		SPIRITS	
	2015	**2017**	**2015**	**2017**	**2015**	**2017**
Daily	14.7	13.9	5.4	7.4	0.6	1.6
5-6 days a week	2.7	2.8	2.4	2.2	0.2	0.3
3-4 days a week	3.0	2.6	3.5	3.6	0.5	0.7
1-2 days a week	10.4	7.9	14.5	10.4	5.1	2.7
2-3 days a month	3.1	4.6	5.0	5.8	2.8	2.3
1 day a month	4.1	3.5	4.8	4.2	4.9	3.0
6-11 days a year	5.1	3.2	5.1	3.1	3.3	2.7
2-5 days a year	10.4	4.5	8.7	2.9	11.6	5.3
1 day in the last 12 months	2.8	1.8	3.9	1.1	3.2	1.7
Never or more than 12 months ago	43.5	55.2	46.8	59.4	67.8	79.8

Source: RARHA 2015 and INPG 2017.

Turning the data on frequency of consumption in the last year into an indicator of the number of days of consumption in a year, we observe that in 2015, on average, consumption occurred during almost five months (144 days), with half of consumers drinking for around two and a half months (78 days). In 2017 the average rises to 165 days. This trend is mainly seen for wine consumption, which takes place on an average of 163 days in the year. Beer consumption takes place during an average of four months (127 days) and spirits consumption almost two months (57 days).

Table 8-10. Number of days in last year on which any alcoholic beverage, wine, beer and spirits is consumed (for the consuming population). (Population aged 15-64) RARHA 2015 and INPG 2017

	Mean	Median	Standard deviation
RARHA 2015			
Any alcoholic beverage	144	78	151
Wine	139	78	154
Beer	91	30	120
Spirits	30	7	62
INPG 2017			
Any alcoholic beverage	165	78	153
Wine	163	78	158
Beer	127	78	138
Spirits	57	12	105

Source: RARHA 2015 and INPG 2017.

Quantity of alcoholic beverages consumed (2015 and 2017)

Another indicator of consumption, besides prevalence and frequency, is the amount of alcohol consumed. Because of its nature and variability, and because it calls for more precise recall by respondents, this is a more difficult indicator to quantify. It can be broken down into several types of information. In both RARHA and INPG, there is a question about the quantity of alcohol consumed (BSQF measure) and two other questions give us information about alcohol volume: one about the average maximum amount of alcohol by volume consumed on a single occasion, and the other about the amount on a risky occasion (risky single-occasion drinking).

The average maximum amount of alcohol consumed on the same occasion provides information on the maximum limit, both for regular and occasional drinking. The results below show that the average maximum volume in Portugal is around 30g among drinkers.

Table 8-11. Average quantity of maximum 100% volume of alcohol in grams consumed on one occasion

	Mean of maximum amount	Mean of normalised maximum amount *
RARHA 2015	33.08	32.89
INPG 2017	32.20	31.87

*Amount excluding outliers
Source: RARHA 2015 and INPG 2017.

Information on average annual drinking volume is given using the BSQF measure, used for three types of alcoholic beverages to estimate alcohol consumption and explore drinking patterns:

- Beer: includes all types of beer, but not those with low alcohol content (less than 2%) or without alcohol.
- Wine: also includes champagne, port, sherry, vermouth etc.
- Spirits: includes whisky, cognac, vodka, gin, liqueurs, shot drinks or other local drinks containing more than 30% alcohol.

Taking into consideration the pros and cons of the different time references noted above, the 'last 12 months' indicator was used as it provides a more comprehensive picture of alcohol consumption and creates the opportunity to study the relationships between consumption and associated problems that are unlikely to have occurred in the last 30 days (Dawson 2003).

This measure is constructed based on the frequency of consumption of each of the alcoholic beverages in the past 12 months, with the scale ranging from 'daily' to 'once a year' and including 'never' as the last category. The consumption frequency scale was recalculated for the number of consumption days using the midpoints of the intervals. The distribution of the number of consumption days is not continuous because it is created from a discrete frequency scale. Specifically, it was defined that when the interviewee indicated daily consumption in the last 12 months, the assumed value would be 365; it would be 338 when 5 to 6 days a week was indicated; 182 when 3 to 4 days a week; 78 when 1 to 2 days a week; 30 when 2 to 3 days a month were indicated; 12 when 1 day a month was indicated; 7 when 6 to 11 days a year were indicated; 3 when 2 to 5 days a year were indicated; and 1 when 1 day in the last 12 months was indicated.

To reduce confusion associated with the concept of 'average', the question referred to the 'usual' amount consumed. The respondent was asked about the usual amount of consumption per day, with the opportunity to choose between different consumption units (e.g., 33cl cans/bottles or 50cl cans/bottles).

The algorithm for calculating the key variables related to annual alcohol consumption was as follows: to transform the specific usual amount of alcoholic beverage consumed into centilitres of pure alcohol (100%), the number of units of each alcoholic beverage that the interviewee declared he usually consumes was multiplied by the predefined volume of that beverage unit (e.g. 33cl or 50cl, separately for each beverage). The result of this calculation was then multiplied by the alcohol content (in percentage) of the beverage (separately for each beverage).

The alcohol content was defined as 0.05% for beer, 0.12% for wine and 0.4% for spirits. The calculation then took into account the distribution of this consumption over the 365 days of the year.

Since there are different units of beverage—20cl, 33cl, 50cl and 100cl for beer, 15cl, 37.5l and 75cl for wine and 5cl for spirits—a variable was constructed to measure the amount of alcohol whenever, for the same beverage, the respondent indicated more than one different unit of that beverage.

The standard formula for all alcoholic beverages and drink units is as follows: number of days per year * number of glasses/bottles * capacity of glass/bottle in cl * alcohol content of drink * 1000/365.

Taking into account the use of two different collection instruments, the figures point to different consumption, although the trends remain the same. That is, wine continues to show the highest amounts (183cl in 2015 and 215cl in 2017), followed by beer (172cl in 2015 and 200cl in 2017); the values for spirits are well below these, at less than 30cl (24cl in 2015 and 27cl in 2017). The average annual volume of any alcoholic beverage was, in 2015, around 380cl. This figure, if we consider the excessively high values self-reported by some respondents, rises in 2017 to 443cl. However, if we do not consider them, the average annual volume for any drink remains stable at 374cl.

Table 8-12. Mean annual consumption volume (in cl, 100% alcohol) by type of beverage (population aged 15-64)

	RARHA 2015		INPG 2017	
	Consumption	Normalised consumption*	Consumption	Normalised consumption*
Any alcoholic beverage	380.2	378.5	442.9	373.7
Wine	183.4	181.7	215.1	167.9
Beer	172.5	172.5	200.6	181.5
Spirits	24.3	24.3	27.3	27.2

* Limiting excessively high values to a set maximum value.
Source: RARHA 2015 and INPG 2017.

We now relate the quantity figures to an average daily value on a consumption day. The average daily amount of alcohol is around 3cl in beer and 2cl in wine and spirits in 2015. The trend continues in 2017, with a slight rise for beer. It should be remembered, however, that the frequency of consumption of spirits is much lower than those of wine and beer. Another point to note is the high value of standard deviation in wine consumption in Portugal, which suggests that there is a high heterogeneity of situations among these consumers with regard to quantities consumed on an average day, with the same occurring for beer in 2017.

Table 8-13. Quantity of 100% alcohol in cl on an average consumption day (population aged 15-64)

	Mean	Median	Standard deviation
RARHA 2015			
Wine	2.31	1.20	7.96
Beer	2.82	2.00	3.30
Spirits	2.31	2.00	1.71
INPG 2017			
Wine	2.33	1.20	9.36
Beer	3.15	2.00	7.27
Spirits	2.12	1.20	2.40

Source: RARHA 2015 and INPG 2017.

To estimate overall alcohol consumption, data on habitual consumption (BSQF) and excessive consumption (RSOD) are combined.

Calculating alcohol consumption in litres, the annual average rose from 4.20 to 5.0 between 2015 and 2017 in the total population; and from 5.9 to 8.5 in the consuming population. Despite the different nature of the two collection instruments, the values are close for the total population.

Table 8-14. Average annual alcohol consumed in litres (in 100% pure alcohol, for total population and consuming population)

	Total population	Consuming population
RARHA 2015	4.2	5.9
INPG 2017	5.0	8.5

Source: RARHA 2015 and INPG 2017.

Risky single-occasion drinking (RSOD) / episodic heavy drinking / binge drinking (2015-2017)

Risky single-occasion drinking (RSOD) was defined, in both surveys, as the consumption of at least 60 grams of 100% alcohol by men on the same occasion and at least 40 grams of 100% alcohol by women.

There are two problems related to the RSOD method: the first concerns the concept of standard drink, when there is no standard drink, with several different ones can be consumed on the same occasion, so having to choose one may not be easy for consumers; the second problem has to do with the concept of occasion, which is imprecisely defined (it can range from a gathering with colleagues after work to a three-day party, with high intakes of different alcoholic drinks in different settings).

In both questionnaires, the question was formulated in the same way: "Over the past 12 months, how often have you consumed six or more alcoholic drinks on a single occasion? For example, how often have you consumed six 25cl glasses of beer, or six 10cl glasses of wine, or six 3cl glasses of spirits or distilled beverages?" (question put to men; the question for women refers to four or more drinks).

In 2015 binge experiences in the last 12 months were reported by 9.8% of consumers, while in 2017 the figure was 10.5%. Daily or almost daily consumption increased from 2015 to 2017 (from 0.3% to 1.0%), while weekly binge consumption decreased (from 2.2% to 1.7%). Monthly binges, the figure for which was 2.3% in 2015, saw this rise to 2.9% in 2017, while binges less frequent than monthly remained at 4.9% in 2015 and 2017.

Subjective drunkenness (2015 and 2017)

The question on intoxication in the RARHA questionnaire was as follows: "How many times in the past 12 months did you drink enough to feel unsteady or with slurred speech?" The word drunkenness was not used in the wording of the question, taking into consideration its cultural sensitivity, at least in some countries, as well as translation challenges. For analytical purposes, the frequency of intoxication was explored using a standard frequency scale converted to the number of days when intoxication was reported.

In the 2016/17 INPG, on the other hand, it was decided to use two questions regarding intoxication. One was formulated as follows: "In the past 12 months, how often did you get drunk (feel unsteady, with slurred speech, vomiting and/or forgetting afterwards what had happened, for example)?"; and the other: "In the past 12 months, how often did you drink until you were 'merry'?"

The reported situations of intoxication mostly happened more than a year ago. Daily intoxications and those on a weekly basis decreased between 2015 and 2017.

Table 8-15. Frequency of intoxication

	RARHA 2015	INPG 2017	
		a)	b)
Daily	1.0	0.4	0.4
5-6 days a week	0.2	0.0	0.3
3-4 days a week	0.5	0.2	0.5
1-2 days a week	1.0	0.3	1.9
2-3 days a month	0.8	0.9	2.6
1 day a month	1.0	1.3	3.4
6-11 days a year	1.4	0.5	3.9
2-5 days a year	4.0	2.6	8.6
1 day in the last 12 months	3.1	3.6	6.0
More than 12 months ago	87.0	90.1	72.4

a) In the last 12 months, how often have you been drunk (e.g. staggered, had difficulty speaking, vomited and/or could not remember afterwards what happened)?; b) In the last 12 months, how often did you drink until you were "merry"?
Source: RARHA 2015 and INPG 2017.

Unrecorded alcohol (2015 and 2017)

The business of illegal drinks is global and in Portugal generates millions of euros every year. Some researchers point out the fact that estimates of alcohol consumption only take into account recorded alcohol, even though there is significant, if not equivalent, production and consumption of unrecorded alcohol.

As we have seen before, it is necessary to bear in mind that figures for recorded alcohol are limited and underestimated because production and consumption outside commercial circuits are ignored. This underestimation is difficult to quantify because a substantial portion of beverage production is not declared, and it is estimated that there are about the same number of producers formally declaring their wine production as those who do not (Pinto 2001; Carvalho 2003).

The WHO estimate of per capita unrecorded alcohol consumption for Portugal from 1995 onwards, for the population aged 15 and over, is 1.0 litre[61]. Also according to the WHO, the estimated value of unrecorded alcohol for the years 2015-2017 (average) was 2.1 litres, equal to that estimated for 2003-2005 and slightly higher than in 2008-2011 (1.9 litres).

The question added in RARHA on this topic allowed there to be a reference value for Portugal, based on self-declarations by the population, of undeclared alcohol acquired (which is different from the consumption of unrecorded alcohol, as there may be some acquisition without consumption).

In 2015, 10.1% of respondents said that they had purchased unrecorded alcohol in the last 12 months, mostly from a domestic source (family members, neighbours or acquaintances who produce and/or make available or sell — 9.0%). In addition to the importance of home-produced alcohol, the much lower percentage weight of those who purchased alcohol outside their country of origin should be noted (1.7%). In 2017 the figures decrease, with 3.5% of respondents saying that they have purchased unrecorded alcohol in the last 12 months: 3.2% did so from domestic sources and only 0.5% from abroad.

---

[61] Source: http://www.who.int/substance_abuse/publications/en/portugal.pdf.

Table 8-16. Percentage of respondents who acquired unrecorded alcohol

	RARHA 2015	INPG 2017
From abroad	1.7	0.5
Domestic	9.0	3.2
Total	10.1	3.5

Source: RARHA 2015 and INPG 2017.

It is home-produced wine, rather than wine purchased outside the country or other types of drink from any source, that has the most significant weight in the percentage of individuals who purchased unrecorded alcohol in Portugal; the 2017 figures are lower than those of 2015.

Table 8-17. Unrecorded alcohol by type of beverage and source (%)

	RARHA 2015	INPG 2017
From abroad		
Spirits	0.9	0.3
Wine	0.8	0.2
Beer	0.3	0.2
Domestic		
Spirits	2.2	1.1
Wine	7.6	2.7
Beer	0.3	0.2
Total		
Spirits	2.9	1.2
Wine	7.6	2.7
Beer	0.6	0.2

Source: RARHA 2015 and INPG 2017.

The calculation presented below takes into account the volume of alcohol indicated in declarations of purchase, considering only its distribution within the group of those who claimed to have purchased it.

Table 8-18. Average volume (in litres) of unrecorded alcohol per individual who reported purchasing unrecorded alcohol

	RARHA 2015	INPG 2017
From abroad		
Spirits	2	9
Wine	2	51
Beer	2	8
Domestic		
Spirits	10	12
Wine	180	90
Beer	2	19
Total		
Spirits	9	12
Wine	179	87
Beer	2	13

Source: RARHA 2015 and INPG 2017.

It should be noted that the data point to quite different values, which is difficult to justify considering that only two years separate the two surveys—a short period of time for such a significant change in behaviours—and that the generation effect is not even felt. This, we believe, reinforces the need for a more careful reflection on methodological issues, such as the design and size of the sample, the size of the questionnaire, the sequence and location of the questions defined, among other aspects that may be considered. This means that the extrapolation of both results to national indicators of consumption quantities, and therefore their extrapolation to the universe, becomes delicate, if not abusive. However, various analyses based on both results, such as the definition of prevalence and consumption profiles, will be valid and reliable readings and, in that sense, more interesting in sociological terms.

Scales for measuring the consequences of consumption

According to the WHO (WHO 2000), the threshold of what is considered hazardous consumption is generally based on scientific criteria and may reflect national strategies for what is considered moderate consumption. In general, the measurement of problematic or risky consumption in substance use questionnaires tends to be based on amount of alcohol ingested, but also using scales or tests built for this purpose. One of the problems related to the indicator of problematic drinking seems to be the existence of several concepts associated with it—dependence, harmful drinking, problematic drinking, among others—each of which presents its own subtle distinctions, both in medical and social terms.

In the context of the classification of alcohol-related problems, the WHO considers the categories of hazardous consumption, harmful consumption and dependence. Although not part of the initial ICD-10 (International Classification of Diseases) classification (WHO 1992), the concept of hazardous consumption was created and introduced by Babor and colleagues: this type of consumption corresponds to a level or pattern of consumption whose persistence increases the likelihood of health harms (Babor et al. 1994). The WHO proposes a working definition of this hazardous behaviour, describing it as an average regular daily consumption of 20g to 40g of alcohol for women, and 40g to 60g for men. Harmful drinking is defined as a pattern of alcohol consumption that causes harm to individuals' health, both physical and mental (WHO 2004). The WHO working definition considers harmful drinking an average regular daily consumption of more than 40g of alcohol in women, and more than 60g per day in men. Alcohol dependence is defined by a set of physiological, cognitive and behavioural phenomena that may develop after repeated consumption of alcohol. It includes an intense desire to consume alcoholic beverages, lack of control over consumption, continued consumption regardless of the consequences, prioritisation of consumption over other activities and obligations, increased tolerance to alcohol, and withdrawal symptoms when consumption is discontinued.

Given that there are many individual and social consequences of excessive alcohol consumption (mortality, disability due to accidents and illnesses, lack of productivity at work, and violence in the family and in crime, among others), it is necessary to identify hazardous and harmful consumption.

However, there is still no standardised comparative research methodology in the European Union to measure the prevalence of alcohol consumption or of excessive consumption, binge drinking or abuse and dependence, even after projects such as SMART[62] and RARHA[63].

The World Health Organization put alcohol on its public agenda as early as the 1980s and has regularly developed valid systems and universal tools. The development of diagnostic criteria and corresponding instruments to operationalise these criteria has a long and complicated history, which we shall not deal with here (see Hasin 2003). According to Bloomfield, Hope and Kraus (2013), currently three measures tend to dominate population-based studies of alcohol: the CIDI-SAM, the AUDADIS and the AUDIT. Having all been developed around the same time, only CIDI and AUDIT were intended for international comparative use (Bloomfield, Hope and Kraus 2013).

With several scales and questionnaires available, the choice of these depends on what is to be assessed. There are tests designed to detect alcohol dependence and others designed to measure hazardous or harmful alcohol consumption. The choice should take into account factors such as: the period to be evaluated (do you want information about recent drinking patterns, lifetime consumption or chronic consumption?); the target population (general population or young population, for example); how the test will be administered (paper and pen or computer?); who will administer the test (self-completion or questions that can be asked by an interviewer or health professional?); etc. Not being diagnostic instruments, brief alcohol consumption questionnaires are aimed at people who could potentially have harmful consumption or dependence.

According to Wallace (2001), the best questionnaires consist of a combination of simple measures of the quantities and frequency of alcohol consumption, one or more questions to identify binge drinking and a few questions to reveal signs of dependence and/or harmful effects of alcohol consumption. Most of the tests present some degree of error. The accuracy

---

[62] SMART — Standardizing Measurement of Alcohol Related Troubles. One of the objectives of this project financed by the European Commission was to develop standardized comparative research methodology on excessive consumption, binge drinking, intoxication, consumption contexts and alcohol dependence (Moskalewicz and Sieroslawski 2010, 4).

[63] One of the work packages had as its objective strengthening the monitoring of consumption patterns and alcohol related harms in Europe (Moskalewicz, Room and Thom 2016, 8).

and reliability of tests are measured and compared according to sensitivity (measures the ability of a test to identify at-risk or dependent drinkers in a population) and specificity (measures the ability of a test to correctly identify individuals who are not hazardous drinkers). The most accurate and reliable tests have high sensitivity and specificity. The fact that tests have a degree of error does not prevent them from being an essential tool in the detection, prevention and also treatment of harmful alcohol consumption.

Without intending to produce an exhaustive review of the existing instruments, which would be beyond the scope of this text, we will highlight those used in our studies and the results obtained.

CAGE[64]

The CAGE test developed in 1968 by Ewing (1984) is very simple and consists of four questions: 1) Have you ever felt you should cut down on your drinking? 2) Have people close to you ever annoyed you by criticizing your drinking? 3) Have you ever felt guilty about your drinking? 4) Have you ever taken alcohol on waking up, to steady your nerves or to get rid of a hangover? Only two of these questions need a positive response from the respondents for them to be considered dependent. This test was designed to identify dependent alcohol consumers and focuses on lifetime consumption rather than current consumption. It was validated in 1974 and is the most widely used test in clinical practice (Smart et al. 1991). It is quick to apply (about 1 minute) and easy to administer. Sensitivity ranges between 60% and 90% and specificity between 40% and 95%. One of the problems pointed to with the use of CAGE is that it does not measure the frequency of alcohol use, drinking levels and binge drinking, all of which are considered factors that may identify individuals in the early stages of problematic consumption (Nilssen and Cone 1994). In the INPG we obtain this information through other questions.

In the 2017 INPG, and according to CAGE, 1.7% of the respondents evidenced alcohol abuse or dependence (as we have seen previously, in the latter test positive responses to two out of four questions is enough to consider that dependence exists).

---

[64] CAGE is the acronym for *Cut down*, *Annoyed by criticism*, *Guilty* and *Eye-opener*.

AUDIT (Alcohol Use Disorders Identification Test)

In 1989, the WHO created AUDIT, which has been validated in several countries, including Portugal (Cunha 2002 apud Jorge et al. 2017). This questionnaire makes it possible to detect different levels of consumption (hazardous use, harmful use and dependence) in a quick and simplified way. Questions 1 to 8 of the questionnaire allow responses expressed on a scale from 0 to 4 points, and answers to questions 9 and 10 range between 0, 2 and 4 points. Use of the original AUDIT found a sensitivity of 97% and a specificity of 78% for hazardous drinking, and a sensitivity of 85% and a specificity of 85% for harmful drinking when a cut-off point greater than or equal to 8 was used (Saunders et al. 1993). AUDIT had good discrimination in a variety of settings but is best suited for the detection of hazardous and harmful use.

In addition to the good psychometric qualities demonstrated in several studies (namely Cunha's study for Portugal), the instrument is easy to apply (in being quick to fill in) as well as to rate and interpret.

AUDIT C (Bush et al. 1998), which includes only the first three quantification questions of the original test, was designed to identify hazardous and harmful consumption in a primary health care setting. The first question is about frequency of consumption; the second is about the amount of alcohol on a typical day of consumption; and the third is about the frequency of episodes of heavy consumption. Men whose AUDIT C score is 5 or higher and women whose score is 4 or higher must complete all 10 items of the AUDIT for a more complete assessment.

With AUDIT, therefore, the higher the score (ranging from 0 to 40), the higher the probability that the individual's alcohol consumption is affecting their health and safety and that he or she has an alcohol dependence: no hazardous consumption (0 points), low-risk consumption (1 to 3 points for women and 1 to 4 points for men), medium-risk consumption (4 to 7 for women and 5 to 7 for men), high-risk or harmful consumption (8 to 19 points) and dependence (20 to 40 points).

The test was applied to the population (aged 15-64) of lifetime consumers in the 2017 INPG, but for the purpose of possible national and international comparisons, a filter was used for the population consuming in the last year. Making use of AUDIT C, excessive consumption in the general population in Portugal stands at around 15%, while 45% of the population is characterised by low-risk consumption. Using the full version of AUDIT, 5% of the population are risk-free, 38% are low risk and 12.5% are medium risk. High-risk drinkers account for 3% of the total population and dependent consumers make up less than 1% of the total population.

RAPS (*Rapid Alcohol Problems Screen*)

RAPS is a brief instrument for screening purposes (Cherpitel 2000). It consists of four simple questions that indicate symptoms of dependence, requiring only one item to be answered positively.

In RARHA 2015, the original RAPS was expanded by including questions on the frequency of these symptoms (1 or 2 times and 3 or more times). The RAPS scale thus made it possible in RARHA 2015 to assess how many symptoms are manifested and how often they occur. To the question "Has anyone told you about things you did or said while drinking that you did not remember?" 4% of the total population answered in the affirmative. Not being able to do what is expected or feeling guilty about one's consumption is mentioned by 2.8% and 1.9% of the total population respectively, and 1.2% say they have a drink first thing in the morning after waking up. Most respondents reported experiencing the symptoms in question only once or twice in the past 12 months, with the exception of having a drink first thing in the morning after waking up (where responses ranged from once or twice to three times or more in the last 12 months). The percentage of those indicating at least one of the symptoms was 3.8%.

CIDI (*Composite International Diagnostic Interview*)

The gold standard recommended by the WHO Collaborative Project on Identification and Management of Alcohol-Related Problems in Primary Health Care is the Composite International Diagnostic Interview (CIDI), developed by the WHO, the National Institute on Alcohol Abuse and Alcoholism (NIAA), the National Institutes of Health (NIH) and the National Institute of Mental Health (NIMH).

The CIDI classifies psychiatric disorders according to ICD-10 and DSM-IV and has been used as an international epidemiological tool in a wide range of socio-cultural settings, showing good reliability and validity (Nelson et al. 2001; Wittchen 1991, 1994; Robins et al. 1989).

The block of questions from CIDI was used in the RARHA 2015 study as an additional diagnostic tool, consisting of 16 symptomatic questions, five of which could be considered as indicators of individual negative consequences of alcohol consumption. This structured interview makes it possible to detect individuals with hazardous and dependent consumption, according to the diagnostic criteria defined by ICD-10 and DSM-IV.

The data can be divided into four groups: individual consequences, physical dependence, loss of control and continued use despite the existence of problems.

Regarding the physical consequences, the following are considered: having little time to do anything else, reducing important activities, having arguments because of consumption, finding it interferes with work, being physically injured/hurt and having been detained by the police. These physical consequences are stated by 1% to 2% of respondents in the RAHRA 2015 study.

As indicators of physical dependence, the following aspects are considered: feeling a strong need to drink, having a higher tolerance for the same amount, and having withdrawal symptoms and consuming in order to avoid those symptoms — all with percentages around 1%.

Compared to the previous groups of questions, loss of control shows higher percentage values, ranging from 1% to 3%; consumption until unintentionally intoxicated is the indicator with the highest number of affirmative answers.

The last block of questions, on continued consumption despite the existence of problems, indicates that almost 1% of the surveyed population continued to consume alcoholic beverages despite serious or recurrent problems caused by them to family members, friends, neighbours or work colleagues, and that 0.5% continued to consume alcohol despite the existence of serious physical or psychological problems.

Thus, taking into account the four scales used in the INPG and RARHA studies and everything that has already been said about the differences between the two studies and the differences between the scales themselves, we do not find strange the difference between the very low value for dependence, at less than 1%, according to the AUDIT test, and the value of less than 4% found by the RAPS test.

It is also worth mentioning that a meta-analysis of peer-reviewed articles on instruments for screening excessive consumption published in English-language journals between 1985 and 1998, with a comparison with the gold standard, concluded that the most effective questionnaires are AUDIT and CAGE, which proved to be feasible, sensitive, specific screening instruments with high positive and negative predictive value, with a power of response and interpretation (Aertgeerts 2001).

Conclusions

We have limited ourselves in this section to questions that may be raised by the measurement of prevalence of alcohol use. Similar problems arise with the measurement of prevalence for other substances that we have not included here, because they involve different specificity and technical treatment cultures.

As we have seen, estimates of alcohol consumption can indeed be made taking into account different perspectives, purposes and methodologies. It is probable that any of the measures—always within their own limits and possibilities, and notwithstanding problems of a more technical nature—can in itself contribute to producing knowledge necessary to support public health policy decisions. However, in seeking to compare different results, this may only be done taking into account the conditions of their production, due to the major threats to their validity and comparability (WHO 2000; Gmel and Rehm 2004; Rehm et al. 2007).

We have seen that, following the same methodology—that of population-based surveys—and keeping the same Research Team, two instruments—the RARHA and the INPG—can produce data that are convergent but with some differences in their amplitudes. These differences are due, in the first place, to the respective international frameworks of each of the instruments, which require specific formatting for the international comparison purposes that are their aim; in addition, these are surveys with different ambitions in terms of their sample sizes — 1,500 in the case of the RARHA and between 12,000 and 15,000 in the case of the INPG. In fact, some comparisons between the two studies are possible because we have created additional conditions for this.

According to the WHO formulation, there are several important purposes for which international and national data on alcohol consumption patterns and levels of alcohol-related problems can be used. In each case, it is important to consider which types of data are best for each purpose. The main distinctions should be between using data to estimate the magnitude of problems over a given time period and the direction of change over a period of time. An additional consideration is the extent to which data sets used for either purpose can also be used to compare prevalence and estimates of similar trends from other countries (WHO 2000).

We can also speak of complementarity with respect to the different indicators mentioned here, and in some cases detailed, according to the purposes pursued or the professional or institutional sensitivities of the users. Taken together, these indicators can design the different solutions to produce knowledge about the problems associated with alcohol consumption, or even about the public policy guidelines related to them, which have increased significantly, as stated in the Global Status Report on Alcohol and Health (2018, 28).

We have presented the main characteristics and missions of the institutions framing the studies, as well as the main producers of information. We also detailed the specifications linked to each measure and their potential and limits.

Despite the divergences and differences, when we discussed the results provided by the different sources using the most varied indicators, we found convergence in terms of the structure of consumption and its trends.

All in all, it seems appropriate to follow the orientation proposed by the aforementioned International Guide for Monitoring Alcohol Consumption and Harm, which deems important the principle of "triangulation" between different data sources, since each producer has its own sources of bias and error (2000, 63).

Given that the monitoring of trends in patterns of alcohol consumption and related problems is fundamental to the evaluation of alcohol policies and preventive interventions, it is important to understand what can be measured, how, and for what purposes. We share the view of Sordo et al. when they state that "there is still much empirical work to be done to improve estimates of per capita alcohol consumption" (2016, 1). Based on what we wrote above, we would say that in order to improve estimates of per capita alcohol consumption, many of the dimensions that are associated with them (from alcohol purchases by international visitors, through alcohol waste and/or spillage and unrecorded alcohol, to the volume and alcohol content of standard drinks...) should be further clarified. Probably, given changing patterns of supply and consumption, and their diversity at the global level, they should be clarified on an ongoing basis.

PART IV

METHODOLOGY OF SURVEY OF GENERAL POPULATION IN PORTUGAL

Presentation

The national survey on drug use among general population (INPG) are carried out by NOVA FCSH[65] for SICAD (General Directorate for Intervention on Addictive Behaviours and Dependencies)[66], with editions in 2001, 2007, 2012 and 2016/17 and a new one underway during 2021.

Having dealt with the issues relating to the social and political contextualisation of the study, as well as its epistemological and methodological implications, the focus in this section is on the technical issues associated with the development of the questionnaire and its application:

- in chapter nine, we shall present the objectives and provide a general framework for the questionnaire;
- in chapter ten, we shall discuss the sampling and survey methodology; and
- in chapter eleven we shall present the structure of the issues addressed.

---

[65] The first study was carried out by CEOS — Investigações Sociológicas, which originated a new centre named CESNOVA — Centro de Estudos de Sociologia da Universidade NOVA de Lisboa, and then CICS.NOVA — Interdisciplinary Centre of Social Sciences, NOVA FCSH. Despite the different names of the research centres, the coordination of the study was always done by Prof. Casimiro Balsa and the research team has been the same in the last three studies.

[66] The initial request was made by the then IDT — Institute on Drugs and Drug Addiction.

CHAPTER 9

PRESENTATION OF OBJECTIVES AND INTERNATIONAL AND INSTITUTIONAL FRAMEWORK

National and international and international context of INPG on drug use

Surveys to characterise the prevalence of drug use in the general population already have a long tradition in Canada and the United States, where these studies have been known since 1960. In European countries the most consolidated experiences are located in the United Kingdom and Scandinavian countries, due in part to the development of their health systems, but these exercises have tended to spread to all European Union countries since the 1990s, according to a systematisation compiled by François Beck (Beck 2006).

The INPG in Portugal, under the circumstances described above, made it possible to respond decisively to the need to overcome the deficit of knowledge and scarcity of data identified in the first version of the National Drug Strategy, with the re-edition of the study since then continuing to meet these needs.

Until the first Survey of the general population was carried out in 2001, Portugal had no experience with this type of exercise, and was one of the last European Union countries to start collecting it. The INPG is one of the indicators promoted by the European Monitoring Centre for Drugs and Drug Addiction. For this reason, the study also fits with the objectives of international comparison that were at the basis of the creation of that European observatory (EMCDDA 1997).

There were, however, studies aimed at specific populations, such as the following[67]:

- surveys on problematic use[68];
- a prison survey, with the first national study carried out by the Drugs Planning and Coordination Bureau in 1988/90 on a representative sample of the population of Portuguese central prisons[69];
- school surveys, which have been conducted since 1987 (Rodrigues 1992), and the ESPAD — European School Survey Project on Alcohol and Other Drugs;
- a survey of minors under the guardianship of the Ministry of Justice (feasibility study in 1991/92 and carried out in 1993) (Rodrigues 1992);

---

[67] For more information, consult Balsa, C., Farinha, T., Urbano, C. and Francisco, A. 2003. *Inquérito Nacional ao Consumo de Substâncias Psicoativas na População Portuguesa 2001*. Lisbon: IDT — Instituto da Droga e da Toxicodependência.

[68] "Inquérito nacional aos indivíduos em tratamento nos centros de atendimento a toxicodependentes" (Freire 1997).

In 1997, in the context of a project undertaken by the EMCDDA to compare estimates of prevalence of heroin use at local level, a study was carried out to estimate prevalence in the city of Setúbal. For this purpose, samples from two different sources—health centres and a care centre for drug addicts—were used. The estimate for the number of individuals with problematic heroin use in that city, after performing a log-linear analysis on the data collected through the capture-recapture method, was 1.82% (population aged 15 to 54). An attempt to improve this calculation (Godinho, Costa and Padre-Santo 1998), using a larger number of samples and a longer period of time (adding data from Setúbal District Hospital and the Public Security Police, which in the original study could not be collected), gave the extremely high result of 4.07%. The authors attribute this value to the fact that one of the essential conditions of this collection method was not respected: guaranteeing that there are no "entries" and "exits" in the population.

See also Jorge Negreiros, *Estimativas de Prevalências e Padrões de Consumo Problemático de Drogas em Portugal*, IPDT, Lisbon, unpublished, relative to 2001.

[69] Negreiros, Jorge. 1997. *Droga-Crime: Estudos Interdisciplinares (volume 4); Consumo de drogas nas prisões portuguesas*. Lisbon: Gabinete de Planeamento e de Coordenação do Combate à Droga, 61 pp.

Torres, Anália Cardoso; Gomes, Maria do Carmo. 2002. *Drogas e Prisões em Portugal*. Lisbon: CIES/ISCTE.

- surveys in a university setting or conducted in delimited places (leisure areas)[70]; and
- the first national survey, conducted in 1983 among young people aged between 12 and 22 (with 2,895 interviews),[71] this based on a questionnaire applied to a national sample of probabilistic type, and which inquired in a detailed way about a wide range of substances commonly considered as drugs.

In the school environment, after the first experiments in 1987 and 1990, in Portugal, two surveys were carried out in 1995 among the student population: one survey was applied to pupils in their 7th, 8th and 9th years of schooling, and the other to pupils in their 10th, 11th and 12th years, both carried out in public secondary schools. In that same year, and in line with a European commitment, Portugal joined the ESPAD — European School Survey Project on Alcohol and Other Drugs group and, within the scope of that programme, the school survey was carried out again in 1999 and 2001[72] and has been conducted regularly since.

The Ministry of Health carried out its three national health surveys in 1987, 1995/96 and 1998/99, surveying people aged 10 and over, but the information collected only concerned tobacco and alcohol consumption. More detailed information on these and other substances (even if only on representations of consumption) was episodically collected using an

[70] Mourão, Vitória; Baptista, João Luís; Torgal, Jorge. 2000. *Observatório ao Consumo de Substâncias Lícitas e Ilícitas em Estudantes do Ensino Superior em Portugal: Relatório de 1998*, Lisbon: Centro de Investigação em Saúde Comunitária.
[71] We are referring to a survey questionnaire commissioned by the then Planning and Coordination Office for the Fight against Drugs (Drugs Planning and Coordination Bureau) from a marketing and public opinion research company (Norma).
[72] Hibell, Björn; Andersson, Barbro; Ahlström, Salme; Balakireva, Olga; Bjarnasson, Thoroddur; Kokkevi, Anna; Morgan, Mark. 2000. *The 1999 ESPAD Report: Alcohol and Other Drug Use Among Students in 30 European Countries*. Stockholm: The Swedish Council for Information on Alcohol and Other Drugs, CAN Council of Europe. Co-operation Group to Combat Drug Abuse and Illicit Trafficking in Drugs (Pompidou Group), 362 pp. + 21 (survey).
Feijão, Fernanda and Lavado, Elsa. 2002. *Inquérito Nacional em Meio Escolar 2001: 3.º Ciclo do Ensino Básico, Consumo de drogas e outras substâncias psicoactivas*. Lisbon.

experimental questionnaire of a regional nature that was applied in 1991 with the purpose of preparing the second National Health Survey.

The lack of tradition in this type of study in Portugal at the beginning of the 21st century was thus manifested at various levels. The lack of accumulated knowledge about the Portuguese reality made it difficult to guide the choice of survey issues and to frame the results. Also, with regard to the application of questionnaires, in Portugal's information collection market the level of professionalisation of interviewers was incipient. Only one company, Intercampus, S. A., was available to ensure the large-scale collection required by the study.

In order to substantiate and deepen the questioning, qualitative research was undertaken, as part of which 52 in-depth interviews were conducted with drug users. The information gathered, whose main guidelines were presented above, allowed us to understand the normative and relationship models relating to substances and consumption.

Over the past 20 years, the INPG in Portugal, has made it possible to consolidate our knowledge on the evolution of the prevalence of the use of licit and illicit substances, namely through the construction of consumer profiles, the assessment of the population's perception of risk of certain behaviours and their perception of access to substances, in addition to estimating the prevalence of the use of various licit psychoactive substances (such as tobacco, alcoholic beverages and tranquillisers without prescription) and illicit ones (cannabis, heroin, cocaine, ecstasy, LSD and amphetamines) that have fed the agenda of health policies in Portugal and Europe. New sections on substances have been added to each new edition (such as magic mushrooms, in 2007) and the detail of consumption of different types of alcoholic drinks.

In addition, the concern with addictive substances has been progressively joined by non-substance addictions, such as the problems associated with gambling and internet use. Other developments in the study have been motivated by the priority given to certain social problems, such as alcohol consumption or, more particularly, alcohol in the workplace.

Aims and specific objectives

We can frame the objectives of the INPGs within four major purposes:

- to study consumption prevalence,
- to analyse the main consumption trends over time,
- to aim to study not only the consumption profile, but also that of the consumer, by associating consumption to users' socio-economic characteristics, and
- to produce internationally comparable information.

These purposes are realised in more specific objectives, which can be updated in each of the study's applications:

a) to find out the extent of the phenomenon of the use of addictive substances and addictive behaviours without substances, such as gambling practices, among noninstitutional populations;
b) to identify the different types of users and consumption patterns with regard to the type of substances used and the frequency and continuity/discontinuity of their use, forms of administration, and types of polyconsumption that exist;
c) to detect the relationships between types of users and patterns of consumption and certain relevant psychosociological variables;
d) to find out and interpret the representations that the different segments of the Portuguese population formulate about the consumption and users of psychoactive substances;
e) to identify the contexts, circumstances and modes of different types of consumption;
f) to maintain the objective of creating all the conditions necessary to ensure that the information on the Portuguese population may be comparable over time and with the information available in other European countries;
g) to develop research instruments suited to the methodologies adopted.

CHAPTER 10

INPG SAMPLING AND SURVEY METHODOLOGY

Universe and sample design

As mentioned in the previous chapter, our universe is the population living in mainland Portugal and in the Autonomous Regions of the Azores and Madeira, aged between 15 and 64, in both cases inclusive, in the 2001 and 2007 applications, and aged between 15 and 74 in the last two applications. The decision to set 15 years as the lower age limit requires that, where minors are selected, the interviewer should seek permission from their parents. The age range considered in the Portuguese sample was initially established according to the EMCDDA guidelines and its modification is justified by the need to extend the study to cohorts whose experiences, when young, coincide with consumption cultures and to better understand the use of licit substances, especially alcohol, in the 65-74 age group. Only the population living in family homes is included, excluding the population living in institutions (military, religious, prison, residences for students or the elderly, etc.), the population living in collective establishments (hotels, guest houses, boarding houses, hostels, etc.) and the homeless population.

We saw earlier that the sampling design adopted in the INPG is characterised by multiple stages, stratified by conglomerates, with selection of the primary units (municipalities) and the secondary units (statistical sections) in a proportional random manner. The selection of the final observation units—individuals—is carried out by the systematic drawing of lots in selecting households and using tables of random numbers to select the individuals within the household. It is a highly complex design, based on the existing model in other countries with a long tradition of surveying this issue (Spain, for example) and allowing us to make up for the absence of a survey base covering the entire population (which exists in other countries). The various phases defined make it possible to ensure the greatest possible coverage at municipal level while guaranteeing the greatest possible degree of randomness, from the selection of the geographical areas to be surveyed in each municipality to the final survey unit, which is the individual.

Let us take a closer look at the sampling design procedures.[73]

Regional breakdown of sample and overrepresentation of less populated regions

In order to proceed with the spatial distribution of the total number of interviews to be carried out, the Nomenclature of Territorial Units for Statistics II (NUTS II) is used. This divides the country into seven regions, with a view to ensuring statistical representativeness. Strictly speaking, this requirement leads to seven regional samples: the North, Centre, Lisbon Metropolitan Area, Alentejo, Algarve, Autonomous Region of the Azores and Autonomous Region of Madeira. This is step 0 in defining the sample: estimating the proportion of the resident population aged 15-74 in each region within the national total.

Step 1 of constructing the sample consists in calculating the number of interviews to be conducted in each NUTS II. In this first distribution, 800 interviews are assigned to each region[74], as a way of guaranteeing a minimum number of interviews which does not jeopardise the representativeness of the data at regional level, while at the same time allowing a minimum segmentation of their populations. Subsequently, the remaining interviews are distributed among all the NUTS, this time in proportion to the size of their population. In the final reckoning, in no region will fewer than 950 interviews be held. The NUTs themselves may reinforce the corresponding sample in order to guarantee better coverage of their local diversities. This reinforcement occurred in the Autonomous Region of the Azores.

Let us make this more precise by way of an example: estimating that the total number of interviews to be carried out is 12,000, and knowing that in

---

[73] In the initial definition of our sample design, we benefited from essential collaboration from Professor Jacinto Osuna, who was associated with the design of the INPG in Spain (Osuna Rodrigues 1999).

[74] In 2012, since the sample size was smaller, to ensure representativeness by NUT II, a base value of 650 interviews in each region was ensured.

each NUT II there will be at least 800 (making a total of 5,600 for the seven regions), the remaining 6,400 are distributed proportionally among the seven NUT II according to the weight of the resident population aged 15-74.

It is possible that rounding up to the unit will end up giving a total of one more interview than initially estimated.

Table 10-1. Step 1 of sample construction: calculation of the quantity of interviews for each NUT II

Resident population aged 15-74 by NUT II* place of residence	Population			Number of interviews	
		Proportion	Common base	Remainder	Total
North	2,775,487	0.356	800	2,280	3,080
Center	1,669,768	0.214	800	1,372	2,172
Lisbon	2,108,445	0.271	800	1,732	2,532
Alentejo	520,954	0.067	800	428	1,228
Algarve	324,876	0.042	800	267	1,067
RA Madeira	201,644	0.026	800	166	966
RA Azores	189,829	0.024	800	156	956
TOTAL	7,791,003	1	5,600	6,400	12,001

* Annual estimates of resident population.

Proportional distribution of interviews per sub-region

Once the total number of interviews to be carried out in each of the regions is known, we proceed to distribute them spatially throughout the territory of each one, taking into account the statistical sub-regions (NUTS III). In this step 2, the distribution is made in proportion to the population weight of each sub-region.

Let us take the example of the Alentejo NUT II. Given the number of interviews estimated for this region (1,228) we proceed to distribute the interviews by each NUT III (sub-region) respecting the principle of proportionality.

Table 10-2. Step 2 of sample construction: calculation of quantity of interviews for each NU III (exemple: sub-regions of Alentejo NUT II)

Resident population aged 15-74 by NUT III*place of residence in Alentejo region	Population	Proportion	Number of interviews
Alentejo Litoral	69,108	0.133	163
Alto Alentejo	76,412	0.147	180
Alentejo Central	111,930	0.215	264
Baixo Alentejo	85,726	0.165	202
Lezíria do Tejo	177,778	0.341	419
TOTAL	520,954	1	1,228

* Annual estimates of resident population.

Stratification by number of inhabitants and selection of primary units — municipalities

In order to proceed, in step 3, to the selection of the municipalities, we first introduce a criterion of stratification that takes into account their number of inhabitants. Two different classifications are used in order to take into account the macrocephaly of the metropolitan areas of Lisbon and Oporto, whose population size is not the same in the panorama of Portuguese municipalities and therefore requires a specific treatment. The use of a single classification for the whole country would be inappropriate insofar as, if it were used, many strata would have no representation except in the North and the Lisbon and Vale do Tejo regions. For these two regions, a stratification by municipality with nine strata was used and for the remaining regions a stratification with only five strata.

This stratification is important in order to be able to proceed with the allocation of interviews in each municipality, respecting the unequal distribution of the population, but, at the same time, ensuring a minimum number of interviews in each sub-section to be drawn. This minimum number, which varies between 7 and 12 (for an average of 10 interviews per sub-section), makes it possible for the efforts in terms of human and financial resources to be more balanced. It is also assumed that the municipalities in the same stratum will have similar population characteristics.

These are the classifications by strata:

Table 10-3. Strata for Oporto and Lisbon metropolitan regions

E1 Municipalities with 5,000 or fewer inhabitants
E2 Municipalities with between 5001 and 10 000 inhabitants
E3 Municipalities with between 10 001 and 50 000 inhabitants
E4 Municipalities with between 50 001 and 100 000 inhabitants
E5 Municipalities with between 100 001 and 150 000 inhabitants
E6 Municipalities with between 150 001 and 200 000 inhabitants
E7 Municipalities with between 200 001 and 300 000 inhabitants
E8 Municipalities with between 300 001 and 600 000 inhabitants
E9 Municipalities more then 600 000 inhabitants

Table 10-4. Strata for remaining Portuguese regions

Municipalities with 5,000 or fewer inhabitants
Municipalities with between 5001 and 10 000 inhabitants
Municipalities with between 10 001 and 50 000 inhabitants
Municipalities with between 50 001 and 100 000 inhabitants
Municipalities with between 100 001 and 150 000 inhabitants

We now proceed to classify the municipalities of each region by their respective strata, using their population size as a criterion. It will also be important that, within each stratum, municipalities be ordered according to population size. Once this classification and ordering has been carried out, the next step will be the proportional distribution of the interviews assigned to each sub-region by each of the strata, according to the sum total of the populations of its municipalities.

Table 10-5. Step 3 of sample construction: calculation of quantity of interviews by strata in each sub-region (exemple: sub-regions of Alentejo NUT II)

Sub-region of Alentejo	Resident population 15-74	Total population	< 5,000	5,001-10,000	10,001-50,000	50,001-100,000	100,001-150,000	150,001-200,000	200,001-300,000	300,001-600,000
Lezíria do Tejo	69,108	237,868	0	21,595	158,852	57,421	0	0	0	0
Alentejo Litoral	76,412	93,521	0	0	93,521	0	0	0	0	0
Alto Alentejo	111,930	104,538	32,909	13,935	57,694	0	0	0	0	0
Alentejo Central	85,726	152,299	11,580	38,646	49,645	52,428	0	0	0	0
Baixo Alentejo	177,778	116,332	13,313	41,418	61,601	0	0	0	0	0
TOTAL	520,954	466,690	57,802	93,999	262,461	52,428	0	0	0	0

	Nº interviews	< 5,000	5,001-10,000	10,001-50,000	50,001-100,000	100,001-150,000	150,001-200,000	200,001-300,000	300,001-600,000
Lezíria do Tejo	419	0	38	280	101	0	0	0	0
Alentejo Litoral	163	0	0	163	0	0	0	0	0
Alto Alentejo	180	57	24	99	0	0	0	0	0
Alentejo Central	264	20	67	86	91	0	0	0	0
Baixo Alentejo	202	23	72	107	0	0	0	0	0
TOTAL	582	72	117	327	65	0	0	0	0

Once the number of interviews to be conducted per sub-region and stratum has been determined, the interviews are distributed by the municipalities of each sub-region and, within the municipalities, by the sample points (statistical sections or sub-sections). The number of sample points is defined according to the number of interviews in the municipality, so that in each point there should be, on average, around 10 interviews. Thus, for example, if in a municipality the planned number of interviews is 19, two sample points will be randomly drawn: in one, there will be 10 interviews and in the other, 9.

The distribution of the number of interviews and sample points per sub-region and municipality follows two principles with inverse effects. In the first place, it is important to concentrate the interviews to be carried out in the smallest possible geographical area. To this end, the reference number was set at 10 for the total number of interviews to be carried out in each sample point drawn (in reality, a minimum of 7 and a maximum of 12 interviews was defined, adjusted according to the number of interviews and sample points defined for each municipality). This number (or this interval) has been adopted so as to make the most of the trips made by the interviewers to the selected locations, while limiting the number of interviews so as to avoid the "alarm" effect that may result from surveying a large number of people in small localities/areas.

When the number of interviews in a particular municipality is less than 7, this number is redistributed among the other municipalities in the same stratum, which — since they are in the same sub-region – are assumed to have similar population and, therefore, behavioural characteristics. Secondly, the interviews assigned to each stratum are distributed equally among the municipalities in each stratum, without taking into account the different sizes of their populations, since a proportionality criterion had already been introduced with the creation of the strata.

Let us continue with the example of the Alentejo, taking now the sub-region of Alentejo Central.

Table 10-6. Step 4 of sample construction: calculation of number of interviews per municipality in a sub-region (exemple: Alentejo Central sub-region)

E1 (< 5000)				E2 (5,000-10,000)				E3 (10,000-50,000)				E4 (50,000-100,000)			
MC	Pop. 15-74	Pop. Total	Nº/Mun.	MC	Pop. 15-74	Pop. Total	Nº/Mun.	MC	Pop. 15-74	Pop. Total	Nº/Mun.	MC	Pop. 15-74	Pop. Total	Nº/Mun.
1870708	1,837	2,450	Agreg	1870713	3,806	5,145	11	1870711	7,397	10,015	21	1870705	39,313	52,428	91
1870707	2,976	4,138	10	1870709	4,251	5,828	11	1870712	8,191	11,255	21				
1870701	3,505	4,992	10	1870710	4,669	6,353	11	1870704	8,967	12,728	22				
				1870703	4,889	6,736	11	1870706	11,275	15,647	22				
				1870702	5,060	6,928	11								
				1870714	5,794	7,656	12								
	8 318		20		28,469		67		35,830		86		39,313		91

Selection of secondary units — the sections

Once the number of interviews to be carried out in each municipality is known, we move on to the next step in designing the sample and the last step to be carried out away from the field: the random selection of secondary sampling units (the conglomerates). The division of the country from a statistical point of view, as produced by the INE, segments the larger units, the regions, progressively subdividing them into smaller units, starting with the sub-region, then the municipalities, the parishes and the statistical sections, which are finally subdivided into sub-sections[75]. It is at this level of statistical sub-sections that we proceed to the last stage of sample selection. Statistical sub-sections aggregate, in principle, sets of population of an approximate size. In urban areas, statistical sections correspond to very small areas, sometimes only a few buildings, but in rural areas they may correspond to very large areas, depending on the population density. With the selection of the statistical sub-sections, we are designating the residential spaces where the interviews will be carried out. For the reasons given above, each of these sample points is assigned a reference quota of 10 interviews. Within each municipality, the number of these points was obtained by dividing the number of interviews allocated to it by 10. In the cases in which the reference 10 could not be respected, it was decided to create sample points with a minimum of 7 and a maximum of 12 interviews. Once the number of sections to be selected in each municipality is known, they are drawn. To do so, the dimensions of the respective populations are listed (municipality by municipality) and added cumulatively so that the value in front of the last section on the list corresponds to the total number of inhabitants of the municipality in question. This is then followed by the actual drawing of lots, which is carried out using a simple random number table. With this last process, the first phase of extracting the sample closes.

The planning of the sample then reaches the point where the locations where the interviews will take place are randomly drawn. Once a list of all the sections (or statistical sub-sections) has been drawn up and the number of sample points in each municipality where the survey teams will work has

---

[75] While in the other editions the geographical unit of analysis was the statistical sub-section, in 2012, due to existing constraints related to sample size, in order to guarantee randomness the geographical unit was the statistical section.

been estimated, the territories for each municipality for which geographical maps are requested are listed and the routes for collecting addresses and, with these, the households to be surveyed are defined.

Table 10-7. Step 5 of sample construction: calculation of number of interviews and sample points per municipality in a sub-region (exemple: Alentejo Central sub-region)

Municipality code	Name of municipality	N.º of interviews	N.º of sample points to be drawn
1870701	Alandroal	10	1
1870702	Arraiolos	11	1
1870703	Borba	11	1
1870704	Estremoz	22	2
1870705	Évora	91	9
1870706	Montemor-o-Novo	22	2
1870707	Mora	10	1
1870708	Mourão	Agreg.	
1870709	Portel	11	1
1870710	Redondo	11	1
1870711	Reguengos de Monsaraz	21	2
1870712	Vendas Novas	21	2
1870713	Viana do Alentejo	11	1
1870714	Vila Viçosa	12	1

In addition to the sample points required in each municipality, as many substitute sample points are drawn to avoid difficulties that may arise in the field, namely: a reduced number of households and/or people eligible to answer the questionnaire; difficulties for interviewers in entering the field (for example, due to social tensions at the time, unforeseen circumstances or natural disasters).

Selection of ultimate units — individuals

To start the next phase of the sample drawing process it is necessary to obtain from the INE the cartography corresponding to the approximately 1,200 statistical sections drawn (for a sample of 12,000), so that the spatial delimitation of the sections can be carried out. This delimitation is essential for the next step, which consists in surveying and enumerating all the existing households within each statistical section.

From this point onwards, the procedures involved in the selection of the sample must be perfectly defined and in a way that leaves no room for doubt, since they will be carried out in full by the members of the field teams. For reasons presented above, the procedures used throughout the sample drawing process are conducted in such a way as to deprive the interviewers of any initiative in choosing the statistical sub-sections, households and individuals selected.
Work on the ground begins by sending a fieldworker to each selected statistical section, equipped with a map of the location on a scale that makes it possible to recognise streets, buildings and single-family dwellings (whenever possible, the map is provided on a scale of 1:2000), but above all the boundaries of the selected section.

At this point, the exact number of interviews to be conducted in each section is already known. On site, an exhaustive survey of the dwellings that exist there is carried out and these must be listed and noted down (street name, door number, dwelling number etc.) so that they can be identified by anyone else. At the same time, the information collected is "cleaned" by removing from the list all dwellings not eligible for the sample, such as commercial or office spaces, uninhabited spaces and, if it is possible to obtain this information, all dwellings in which the residents are outside the age limits of the study (15-64/74). Once all the dwellings found have been numbered in ascending order and all information making possible their identification has been recorded, the company responsible for the fieldwork, in cooperation with a member of the research team, will choose the first household to be contacted and the selection interval that will make it possible to choose the households to be contacted next. This systematic selection procedure, to be applied in the field by the interviewer, is controlled so as to eliminate any initiative on the part of the interviewer to circumvent the established selection. Once the households to be contacted have been defined, the final sampling unit—the individual—must be selected. This table is built on the basis of information from the Census on the composition of households and should ensure that the age structure of the sample population reproduces that of Portugal's population. When establishing contact with someone in the selected dwelling, the interviewer should use it to determine which resident will be selected. Only this individual will be able to answer the questionnaire, and it is not possible under any circumstances to substitute another person. The interviewer is not allowed to intervene in the selection process, thus guaranteeing the conditions of randomness that the study requires.

Size of sample

The size of the Portuguese sample has been calculated to ensure a "comfortable" representation of drug users, aiming as far as possible to characterise the profile of this population. Despite this orientation, it is a difficult aim to achieve a very fine characterisation in the case very minority consumption. Since it was not possible to index the size of the sample on very minor use (which would cause it to shoot up to prohibitive values) it was decided to define a theoretical sample that would guarantee a good cost-benefit ratio, taking into account the proposed objectives and the margins of error that could be calculated. The theoretical sample was therefore set at 15,000 individuals in 2001 and 2007, and 7,000 individuals in 2012 (a reduction due to budgetary reasons), with 12,000 individuals in 2016/17.

Table 10-8. Evolution of sample size 2001 to 2016/17 (n)

	2001	2007	2012	2016/17
Population aged 15-64	14,184	12,202	5,355	9,632
Population aged 15-74	--	--	6,817	12,023

Construction of field sample

The fieldwork has encountered the expected difficulties, taking into account the methodology used, the size of the sample and the subject of the study. The very methodology of selecting households, through surveys supported by a cartography of the statistical sections, besides being unusual, has posed additional difficulties due to the fact that the information that is provided by the INE is not always up to date. It has sometimes happened that new residential settlements have perverted the information available for urban statistical sections or, in the case of rural regions, that the expected households are not found. In cases where it is considered that the change in the residential fabric may affect the quality of the sample, the sections in question are replaced by others that were previously drawn as substitutes. A supplementary draw is also made in the case of households. To make the principle of no substitution feasible, more households are selected in advance than need to be contacted for sampling. In addition to non-residential dwellings (offices, shops, etc.) excluded from the draw, there are a number of households that are ineligible, based on the definition of the survey population, where residents are absent or refuse the first contact. Doubling the number of selected households—for each selected section, 20 households are drawn instead of the expected 10—allows the interviewers to proceed with the applications, excluding any intervention on their part in the choice of households. This procedure has allowed the application of the questionnaire in all the defined sample units, with a few exceptions.

The fact that all households to be contacted were selected from the outset, with no substitution taking place in the case of a refusal to answer or absence from the residence, brings an additional difficulty to the fieldwork. Usually, interviewers can substitute people who do not respond or who are not at home with others living in the same area and with profiles that the interviewer considers to be equivalent — so enabling an interviewer to always conduct the number of interviews expected in the place visited. This facility did not exist with the methodology adopted. In fact, if there are no substitutions, the interviewer must return to the dwelling until contact can be established (the decision to consider the home unoccupied can only be made after three attempts and, even then, it has to be validated by information from a duly identified neighbour, as a control). The number of attempts that the interviewer is obliged to make was initially established as three, subsequently changed to as many as possible, to try to reduce the number of cases in which no contact is made.

The complexity of the whole process means that numerous documents have to be produced to control its various phases. In addition to the information provided to interviewers (Fieldwork manual), others are produced that make it possible to verify and monitor interviewers' performance throughout the various phases of the process (household survey, contact with households...).

The fieldwork is verified by two means: checking the consistency of the materials produced by the interviewer and telephone or face-to-face contact with the households where questionnaires are conducted. During the entire period in which the applications are being carried out, a toll-free number based at the research centre is in operation to answer any questions that the people contacted may have. This number is provided in a cover letter distributed to all selected households prior to any personal contact. In most cases people want to confirm the origin of the initiative or the procedures buy which homes were selected.

Conducting interviews

Information was collected through the personal interview method using the CAPI (computer-assisted personal interviewing) system between 2007 and 2016/17; in the first application the questionnaire had been in paper format.

Table 10-9. Data collection periods 2001 to 2016/17

2001	April to July and September to December 2001
2007	January to November 2007
2012	December 2011 to April 2012 (control collection from December 2012 to March 2013)
2016/17	December 2016 to June 2017 (control collection in September 2017)

All fieldwork is organised according to the guidelines defined in a Fieldwork manual, which provides all the forms that must be used to carry out the various operations described in the previous paragraphs.

The interview itself is governed by specific conditions, taking into account the nature of the themes addressed: interviews on consumption require extra care to ensure a good understanding of the information to be collected, but also to guarantee the confidentiality of the responses in cases where someone else may also be in the place where the interview is carried out.

It is thus stipulated in the manual that in the block of questions on illicit psychoactive substances, the interviewer need not mention aloud the names of the substances or the most common terms that designate them; this principle is intended to protect the confidentiality of the information throughout the interview. More specifically:

- The interviewer, when reading the question, should not read out the name of the psychoactive substance (for example: cannabis, hashish, marijuana, liamba, chamon) or any information that is in brackets in the text of the question. There is no need to read this term because on the cards associated with these questions the names of the various substances referred to in the question are always provided.
- In turn, the respondent reads the name of the illicit psychoactive substance on the card and answers the question without having to refer to it out loud. In this way, the interviewer asks all questions by saying "this product", in the way that all questions are formulated.

If, because interviewees are distracted or do not understand how this method works, they ask "what product?" then the interviewer answers: "The product that is written on the card."

Weighting and analysis of data

The analysis should respond fully to the research objectives that were previously defined. Others may, however, emerge in the course of the discovery process itself, when the research "feeds" on itself.

But, before this process, it is important to adjust and correct the data so that they are representative of the general population. For this reason, a weighting of the data is carried out, based on the criteria that were the basis for the construction of the sample itself — in this case, distribution by region (NUT II), gender and age group. The weighting makes it possible to compensate for the various possible causes of imbalance in the sample during the fieldwork.

CHAPTER 11

STRUCTURE OF QUESTIONNAIRE CONTENT

During the five applications of the INPG we tried to maintain the structure of the questionnaire without major changes. On the one hand, there are questions that are formatted line with the need for international comparison. On the other, monitoring consumption trends in the medium term also means that it is not possible to change the collection of certain indicators.

As this is the dominant concern, evidently the questionnaire has been subject to various developments or changes. This necessary adaptation is due to changes in consumer cultures, with the appearance of new substances or new circumstances or modes of consumption; the sensitivity of public policies is also changing, making it necessary to deepen the knowledge of certain behaviours.

As mentioned above, these changes make it difficult to achieve a balance between epidemiological concerns and those with the contextualisation (sociological, psychological...) of consumption, and it is clear that the size of the questionnaire is always difficult for the researcher to manage because it is always too long.

Below we present the themes addressed in the questionnaire used in the 2021 application.

Individual characterisation of respondents

The individual characterisation of respondents is obtained through:

- sociodemographic characterisation;
- socio-economic characterisation;
- experience of schooling;
- professional experience (extended to work-related consumption experience as of the 2012 application); and

- participation in migratory processes.

Characterisation of households

Characterisation of households then completes and contextualises the individual characteristics of the respondents, with information being collected on:

- household structure;
- characterisation of the spouse;
- characterisation of parents/grandparents;
- income, housing and property.

Sociabilities

The survey applications carried out in 2001 and 2007 included a battery of questions on social networks and sociability, focused mainly on friendships, in an attempt to better explore the knowledge of one of the possible aspects of consumption. In the 2012 and 2016/17 applications, the priorities given to the consumption of alcohol and, above all, to alcohol consumption in the workplace, prompted us to exclude the collection of this information on sociability. The occurrence of the crisis caused by the pandemic that started in February 2020, and the need to study its possible effects on consumption, motivated us to reintroduce this battery, adapted to the new circumstances, in the survey conducted in 2021.

Health and relationship with the body

In this block we collected information on indicators used in measurement of alcohol consumption, on experiences of treatment of alcohol problems by health institutions, and on attitudes and representations of risk associated with the consumption of certain substances:

- health care;
- experiences with covid-19/SARS-CoV-2;
- attitudes towards risky behaviours.

Licit psychoactive substances

The licit psychoactive substances studied are the following:

- tobacco;
- alcoholic beverages;
- medicines, sedatives, tranquillisers and hypnotics (benzodiazepines);
- stimulant medicines (nootropics) — from 2021 onwards;
- analgesic medicines (opioids) — from 2021 onwards.

Illicit psychoactive substances

As for illicit substances, the list used in the 2021 application is as follows:

- cannabis (hashish, weed, liamba, marijuana, chamon);
- ecstasy (tablets);
- amphetamines (speed);
- cocaine (coke);
- heroin (powder, horse);
- Relevin;
- LSD (acid);
- magic mushrooms / hallucinogens;
- "new psychoactive substances";
- other substances perceived as drugs.

Representations and perceptions of risk

This block applies batteries of questions suggested by the European Monitoring Centre for Drugs and Drug Addiction to monitor the representations of risks and attitudes associated with the use of certain substances:

- representations;
- risk perceptions.

Non-substance addictions

Non-substance addictions, which have been mainly studied since the application carried out in 2016/17, are the subject of enhanced attention in the 2021 application. The following behaviours are considered:

- gambling;
- gaming;
- internet.

Completion procedures (closing questions)

In this last block, information is collected that makes it possible to manage the interview controls. The credibility that the interviewer attributes to the information collected is also noted.

Reasons for non-responses

An attached questionnaire provides the opportunity to characterise the selected individuals who refused to answer the questionnaire and, if possible, the reasons why they did so.

Pattern of questions for addictive substances and non-substance addictions

Addictive substances

For each substance the same pattern of questions was used as far as possible:

1. Prevalence — lifetime, last 12 months, and last 30 days
2. Pattern — lifetime, last 12 months and last 30 days
3. Quitting
4. Consumption career:
    - 4.1. first time
    - 4.2. usually
    - 4.3. last time
    - 4.4. consumption circumstances

4.5. consumption contexts
4.6. access to substance
4.7. motivations for consumption
5. Mode of consumption
6. Problematic consumption/dependence:
6.1. Richmond and Fagerström tests (tobacco)
6.2. CAGE and AUDIT (alcohol)
6.3. SDS and CAST (cannabis)
6.4. DSM (other substances).

Non-substance addictions (gambling, gaming and internet)

1. Prevalence — lifetime, last 12 months and/or last 30 days.
2. Pattern — lifetime pattern, last 12 months and/or last 30 days.
3. Consumption career.
4. Problematic/dependent behaviour:
4.1. SOGS (gambling)
4.2. Portuguese Internet Gaming Disorder Scale — Short-Form (gaming)
4.3. Internet Addiction Test (internet).

BIBLIOGRAPHICAL REFERENCES

Abraham, M.D., Cohen, P.D.A., de Winter, M.A. L., & van Til, R.-J. 1999. *Licit and Illicit Drug Use in the Netherlands, 1997*. Amsterdam: CEDRO CENTRUM VOOR DRUGSONDERZOEK, UVA.

Adlaf, E.M. 2005. Collecting drug use data from different populations. In Zili Sloboda (ed.), *Epidemiology of Drug Abuse* (pp. 99-111). Springer, Boston, MA.

Aertgeerts, B., Buntinx, F., Ansoms, S., & Fevery J. 2001. Screening properties of questionnaires and laboratory tests for the detection of alcohol abuse and dependence in a general practice population. *British Journal of General Practice*. 51: 206-17.

ALAC. 1996. *Guidelines for Alcohol and Drug Assessment: a review of alcohol and drug screening, diagnostic and evaluation instruments*. Wellington: Alcohol Advisory Council of New Zealand.

Alanko, T. 1984. An overview of techniques and problems in the measurement of alcohol consumption. In Reginald G. Smart, Howard D. Cappell, Frederick B. Glaser, Yedy Israel, Harold Kalant, Robert E. Popham, Wolfgang Schmidt & Edward M. Sellers (eds.), *Research Advances in Alcohol and Drug Problems*, Tom 8 (pp. 209-226). Plenum Press, New York and London.

Andersen, Hans Christian. 2015. *Contos*. Temas & Debates.

Anderson, P., Møller, L., & Galea, G. 2012. *Alcohol in the European Union Consumption, Harm and Policy Approaches*. Edited by World Health Organization. Copenhagen.

Babor, T.F, Campbell, R., Room, R., & Saunders, J. (eds.). 1994. *Lexicon of alcohol and drug terms*. Geneve: World Health Organization.

Balsa, Casimiro. 2002. Les ressources d'une population en situation de grande précarité. In Vivianne Chatel and Marc-Henry Soulet, *Faire face et s'en sortir – Développement de compétences et action collective* (pp. 289-300). Fribourg (Suisse): Res Socialis.

Balsa, C., Farinha, T., Urbano, C., & Francisco, A. 2003. *Inquérito Nacional ao Consumo de Substâncias Psicoactivas na População*

Portuguesa 2001. Coleção Estudos Universidades. Lisboa: Instituto da Droga e Toxicodependência.

Balsa, C., Vital, C., Urbano, C., & Pascueiro, L. 2008. *Inquérito Nacional ao Consumo de Substâncias Psicoactivas na População Geral, Portugal 2007*. Coleção Estudos Universidades. Lisboa: Edição Instituto da Droga e Toxicodependência, IP.

Balsa, C., Vital, C., & Pascueiro, L. 2011. *O consumo de bebidas alcoólicas em Portugal 2001-2007. Prevalências e padrões de consumo*. Lisboa: Instituto da Droga e da Toxicodependência.

Balsa, C., Vital, C., & Urbano, C. 2014. *Inquérito Nacional ao Consumo de Substâncias Psicoativas na População Geral, Portugal 2012*. Lisboa: Serviço de Intervenção nos Comportamentos Aditivos e nas Dependências.

Balsa, C., Vital, C., & Urbano, C. 2018. *IV inquérito nacional ao consumo de substâncias psicoativas na população geral, Portugal 2016/17*. Lisboa: Serviço de Intervenção nos Comportamentos Aditivos e nas Dependências.

Balsa, Casimiro (org.). 2019. *Difração Normativa, Comportamentos Escondidos e Identidades Transversas*. Vila Nova de Famalicão: Edições Húmus e CICS.NOVA.

Balsa, Casimiro (ed.). 2020a. Diffraction normative, comportements cachés et identités transverses. *Res Social*. Schwabe Verlag. https://doi.org/10.24894/978-3-7965-4146-9.

Balsa, Casimiro. 2020b. L'émergence du paradigme interprétatif de la discrétion et des théories sur l'implémentation aux USA. In Marc-Henry Soulet, *Pouvoir discrétionnaire et pratique réflexive – la position paradoxale des « faiseurs » d'action publique*. Basel: Schwabe Verlag.

Balsa, Casimiro. 2022. A construção de espaços de transgressão: o consumo de drogas. In Domingos Vaz & Antônio Dimas Cardoso, *Cidades, Escalas e Transações* (pp. 40-87). Vila Nova de Famalicão: Edições Húmus.

Balsa, Casimiro. 2006. A exclusão e o espaço, espaços de exclusão. In Casimiro Balsa, *Relações Sociais de Espaço – Homenagem a Jean Remy* (pp. 13-33). Lisboa: Colibri/CEOS.

Balsa, C., Urbano, C., & Vital, C. 2021. *O Consumo de Álcool e Outras Drogas pela População Laboral, 2001-2021. Vinte anos de pesquisa sobre o consumo de substâncias psicoativas em Portugal*. Coleção Navegar é Preciso. Vila Nova de Famalicão: Edições Húmus.

Barth, Fredrik. 1998. *Ethic Groups and Boundaries, The Social Organization of Culture Difference*. Long Grove, Illinois: Waveland, Press, Inc.

Beck, François. 2006. *Entre représentativité des échantillons et représentations des usages : l'apport des enquêtes en population générale à la compréhension des usages de drogues*. Université René Descartes – Paris V – Sorbonne.

Beck, F., & Peretti-Watel, P. 2001. Les Usages de drogues illicites déclarés par les adolescents selon le mode de collecte. *Population* 6 (56e année): 963-85.

Becker, Howard S. 1985. *Outsiders, Études de sociologie de la déviance*. Paris: Éditions A.-M. Métailié.

Bellis, M., Hughes, K., Cook, P., & Morleo, M. 2009. *Off Measure: How we underestimate the amount we drink*. Liverpool: Centre for Public Health, Liverpool John Moores University.

Berthelot, Jean-Michel. 1998. *L'Intelligence du social*. Presses Universitaires de France. https://doi.org/10.3917/puf.berth.1998.01.

Beullens, K., Loosveldt, G., Vanderplas, C., & Stoop, I. 2018. Response rates in the European social survey: Increasing, decreasing, or a matter of fieldwork efforts? *Survey Methods: Insights from the Field*. https://doi.org/https://doi.org/10.13094/SMIF-2018-00003.

Bloomfield, K., Hope, A., & Kraus, L. 2013. Alcohol survey measures for Europe: A literature review. *Drugs: education prevention and policy*, 20(5), 348-360. http://dx.doi.org/10.3109/09687637.2011.642906.

Bonevsky, B., Magin, P., Horton, G., Foster, M., & Gisgis, A. 2011. Response rates in GP surveys – Trialling two recruitment strategies. *Australian Family Physician* 40(6): 427-30.

Boniface, Sadie, & Shelton, Nicola. 2013. How is alcohol consumption affected if we account for under-reporting? A hypothetical scenario. *European Journal of Public Health* 23(6): 1076-81. https://doi.org/10.1093/eurpub/ckt016.

Bourdieu, Pierre. 1977. La Censure social. *Science Information, Sage Journals* 16(3-4): 385-88. https://doi.org/10.1177 %2F053901847701600307).

Bush, K., Kivlahan, D.R., McDonell, M.B., Fihn, S.D., & Bradley, K.A. 1998. The AUDIT alcohol consumption questions (AUDIT C): An effective brief screening test for problem drinking. *Archives of internal medicine*. 15:1789-95.

Carvalho, A. 2003. Bebidas alcoólicas: problema de saúde pública. In Maria Isabel Clímaco e Luís Moura Ramos (coord). *Álcool, tabaco e jogo: Do lazer aos consumos de risco* (pp. 137-167). Coimbra: Quarteto.

Castel, Robert. 1995. *Les Métamorphoses de la question sociale une chronique du salariat. L'espace du politique*. Paris: Fayard. http://catalogue.bnf.fr/ark:/12148/cb370186631.

Cherpitel, C.J. 2000. A brief screening instrument for alcohol dependence in the emergency room: The RAPS 4. *Journal of Studies on Alcohol*, 61, 447-449.

http://pubs.niaaa.nih.gov/publications/AssessingAlcohol/InstrumentPDFs/54_RAPS4.pdf.

Christian L.M. 2007. *How Mixed-Mode Surveys are Transforming Social Research: The influence of survey mode on measurement in web and telephone surveys*. Washington State University.

Colliot-Thélène, Catherine. 2006. *La Sociologie de Max Weber*. Paris: Éditions La Découverte.

Dawson, Deborah A. 2003. Methodological Issues in Measuring Alcohol Use. *Alcohol Research & Health*, 27(1): 18-29.

Dawson, Deborah and Robin Room. 2000. Towards agreement on ways to measure and report drinking patterns and alcohol-related problems in adult general population surveys: the SkarpoÈ Conference overview. *Journal of Substance Abuse*, 12: 1-21.

De Leeuw, E. 2005. To mix or not to mix data collection modes in surveys. *Journal of Official Statistics*, 21(2), 233-255.

De Leeuw, E. 2008. Choosing the method of data collection. In De Leeuw, E., Hox, J.J., & Dillman, D., *International Handbook of Survey Methodology*, EAM series (pp. 113-135). New York: Taylor & Francis, Psychology Press.

De Leeuw, E., & Hox, J.J. 2011. Internet surveys as part of a mixed-mode design. In Das, M., Ester, P., & Kaczmirek, L., *Social and Behavioral Research and the Internet*. New York, London: Routledge Taylor & Francis Group, 9.

Dillman, D., Smyth, J.D., & Christian, L.M. 2009. *Internet, mail, and mixed-mode surveys: the tailored design method*. Hoboken, New Jersey: John Wiley & Sons, Inc.

Duffy, B., Smith, K., Terhanian, G., & Bremer, J. 2005. Comparing data from online and face-to-face surveys. *International Journal of Market Research*, Vol. 47, 6, 615-639.

EMCDDA. 1997. *Estimating the Prevalence of Problem Drug Use in Europe*. EMCDDA Scientific Monograph Series N° 1. Lisbon: EMCDDA.

EMCDDA. 2002. *Handbook for Surveys on Drug Use among the General Population – Final report*. Lisboa.

Ewing, J.A. 1984. Detecting alcoholism: the CAGE questionnaire. *JAMA*, 252(14): 1905-1907.

Ferris, J., Templeton, L., Wong, S. 1994. *Alcohol, Tobacco and Marijuana: Use, Norms, Problems and Policy Attitudes among Ontario Adults. A Report of the Ontario Alcohol and Other Drug Opinion Survey, 1992*. ARF Internal Document No. 118, Toronto: Addiction Research Foundation.

Fitzgerald, J.L. 1996. Hidden populations and the gaze of power. *Journal of the Drug Issues* 1(26): 5-21.

Fowler, F. J. 2002. *Survey Research Methods*, 3rd Edition. London: Sage.

Freire, Sofia. 1997. "Estimating the number of opiate use in Setúbal" In EMCDDA. *Final Report – EMCDDA Project: Methodological Pilot Study of Local Level Prevalence Estimates*. Lisbon: EMCDDA

Fricker, Jr., R.D., & Schonlau, M. 2002. Advantages and disadvantages of Internet research surveys: Evidence from the literature. *Field Methods*, 14: 347-67.

Fricker, S., Galesic, M., Tourangeau, R., & Yan, T. 2005. An experimental comparison of web and telephone surveys. *Public Opinion Quarterly*, 69(3): 370-92.

Gameiro, Aires. 2000. *Alcoolismo nos Açores e Madeira: padrões de consumo em 1999 e 2000: linhas de Prevenção*. Lisboa: Hospitalidade.

Gmel, Gerhard, & Rehm, Jürgen. 2004. Measuring alcohol consumption. *Contemporary Drug Problems: An Interdisciplinary Quarterly,* 31(3), 467–540.

Gorman, Emma, Alastair H. Leyland, Gerry McCartney, Ian R. White, Srinivasa Vittal Katikireddi, Lisa Rutherford, Lesley Graham, and

Linsay Gray. 2014. Assessing the Representativeness of Population-Sampled Health Surveys Through Linkage to Administrative Data on Alcohol-Related Outcomes. *American Journal of Epidemiology*, 180(9): 941–948.

Groves, Robert M. 2006. Nonresponse rates and nonresponse bias in household surveys. *Public Opinion Quarterly* 70(5): 646-75. https://doi.org/10.1093/poq/nfl033.

Harkin, A.M. 1995. *Profiles of alcohol consumption in the Member States of the European Region of the World Health Organization*. Copenhague: World Health Organization Regional Office for Europe.

Hasin, D. 2003. Classification of alcohol use disorders. *Alcohol Research and Health* 27, 5-17.

Heckathorn, Douglas. 1997. Respondent-driven sampling: A new approach to study hidden populations. *Social Problems* 44(2): 174-99.

Hoebel *et al.* 2014. Mode differences in a mixed-mode health interview survey among adults. *Archives of Public Health*, 72:46, 1-12.

INE – Instituto Nacional de Estatística. 2012. *Inquérito às Despesas das Famílias 2010-2011*. Lisboa: Instituto Nacional de Estatística, I.P

INE – Instituto Nacional de Estatística. 2014. *Balança Alimentar Portuguesa 2008-2012*. Destaque. Informação à comunicação social. Lisboa: INE.

INE – Instituto Nacional de Estatística. 2017. *Balança Alimentar Portuguesa 2012-2016*. Lisboa: INE.

INE – Instituto Nacional de Estatística. 2017. *Relatório de Atividade do Instituto Nacional de Estatística, IP – 2017*. Lisboa: Instituto Nacional de Estatística, I.P

INE/INSA. 2009. *Inquérito Nacional de Saúde 2005/2006*. Lisboa: INE/INSA.

INE/INSA. 2016. *Inquérito Nacional de Saúde 2014*. Lisboa: INE/INSA.

INSA – Instituto Nacional de Saúde Dr. Ricardo Jorge, Observatório Nacional de Saúde. 2001. *Inquérito nacional de saúde, 1998/1999: dados gerais*. Lisboa: INSA.

INSEE. 2019. *INSEE – rapport d'activité 2019*. Paris. https://rapport-activite.insee.fr/wp-content/uploads/INSEE_RAPPORT_DACTIVITE_2019.pdf.

Johnson, Timothy P. 2014. Sources of error in substance use prevalence surveys. *Hindawi Publishing Corporation, International Scholarly Research Notices* 2014 (Article ID 923290): 21. http://dx.doi.org/10.155/2014/923290.

Jorge, F.M., Moreira, M.T., Pereira, M.O., & Barroso, T. 2017. Intervenções breves na redução do consumo de álcool em utentes de uma unidade de saúde familiar. *Revista de Enfermagem Referência*, vol. IV, 14: 79-87.

Kling, W. 1991. Measurement of ethanol consumed in distilled spirits. *Journal of Studies on Alcohol*, 52(5): 503–504.

Kraus, Florian, & Steiner, Viktor. 1998. Modelling heaping effects in unemployment duration models — With an application to retrospective event data in the German socio-economic panel. *Journal of Economics and Statistics*, 217(5), 550-573.

Krosnick, J.A. 1991. Response strategies for coping with the cognitive demands of attitude measures in surveys. *Applied Cognitive Psychology*, 5(3), 213-236.

Krosnick, J.A., & Alwin, D.F. 1987. An evaluation of a cognitive theory of response – Order effects in survey measurement. *Public Opinion Quarterly*, 51(2), 201-219.

Lachenmeier, Dirk, Gmel, Gerhard & Rehm, Jürgen. 2013. Unrecorded alcohol consumption. In Peter Boyle, Paolo Boffetta, Albert B. Lowenfels, Harry Burns, Otis Brawley, Witold Zatonski, Jürgen Rehm (eds.), Alcohol: Science Policy and Public Health (pp.132-140). Oxford, U.K.: Oxford University Press.

Lavrakas, Paul J. 2013. Applying a total error perspective for improving research quality in the social, behavioral, and marketing sciences. *Public Opinion Quarterly* 77(3): 831-50. https://doi.org/10.1093/POQ/NFT033.

Legleye, Stéphane. 2018. The Cannabis Abuse Screening Test and the DSM-5 in the general population: Optimal thresholds and underlying common structure using multiple factor analysis. *International Journal of Methods in Psychiatric Research* 27(2). https://doi.org/10.1002/MPR.1597.

Legleye, S., Guignard, R., Richard J.-B., Kraus, L., Pabst, A., & Beck, F. 2015. Properties of the Cannabis Abuse Screening Test (CAST) in the general population. *International Journal of Methods in Psychiatric Research* 24(2): 170-83. https://doi.org/10.1002/MPR.1465.

Legleye, S., Piontek, D., Kraus, L., Morand, E., & Falissard, B. 2013. A validation of the Cannabis Abuse Screening Test (CAST) using a latent class analysis of the DSM-IV among adolescents. *International Journal of Methods in Psychiatric Research* 22(1): 16-26. https://doi.org/10.1002/MPR.1378.

Linstone, H.A. and Turoff, M. 1975. *The Delphi: Method: Techniques and Applications*. Reading, MA: Addison-Wesley.

Livingston, Michael e Sarah Callinan. 2015. Underreporting in alcohol surveys: whose drinking is underestimated?. *Journal of Studies on Alcohol and Drugs*, 76(1): 158-64.

Lopes C, Torres D, Oliveira A, Severo M, Alarcão V, Guiomar S, Mota J, Teixeira P, Rodrigues S, Lobato L, Magalhães V, Correia D, Carvalho C, Pizarro A, Marques A, Vilela S, Oliveira L, Nicola P, Soares S, Ramos E. 2017. *Inquérito Alimentar Nacional e de Atividade Física, IAN-AF 2015-2016: Relatório de resultados*. Universidade do Porto. ISBN: 978-989-746-181-1. Disponível em: www.ian-af.up.pt.

Macer, T. 2005. Weaving, not drowning: an update on take-up and best practices in mixed- and multi-mode research. www.meaning.uk.com/resources/articles_papers/files/ spss_directions_2005.pps.

Manthey, J., K. Shield, Margaret Rylett, O. M. Hasan, C. Probst, J. Rehm. 2019. Global alcohol exposure between 1990 and 2017 and forecasts until 2030: a modelling study. *The Lancet*, 393: 2493-2502.

Montonen, Marjatta. 2016. *RARHA Delphi survey: "Low risk" drinking guidelines as a public health measure*. Joint Action RARHA's Work Package 5.

Morgan, David L. 2008. Snowball sampling. *The SAGE Encyclopedia of Qualitative Research Methods. SAGE Publications, Inc.*, 816-17.

Moskalewicz, Jacek and Janusz Sieroslawski. 2010. *Drinking population Surveys – Guidance document for standardized approach. Final report prepared for the project standardizing measurement of alcohol-related troubles – SMART*. Warsaw: Institute of Psychiatry and Neurology.

Moskalewicz, J., Room, R., & Thom, B. (eds.). 2016. *Comparative monitoring of alcohol epidemiology across the EU. Baseline assessment and suggestions for the future action. Synthesis Report*. RARHA work package 4.

Muller, Pierre. 2000. L'Analyse cognitive des politiques publiques : Vers une sociologie politique de l'action publique. *Revue Française de Science Politique*. Sciences Po Les Presses. https://doi.org/10.2307/43119726.

National Institute on Alcohol Abuse and Alcoholism (NIAAA). 2003. *Helping Patients With Alcohol Problems: A Health Practitioner's Guide.* NIH Pub. No. 03–3769. Bethesda, Maryland: NIAAA.

Nelson, C.B., Kessler, R.C., & Mroczek, D. 2001. *Scoring the World Health Organisation's Composite International Diagnostic Interview short form*. Geneva: World Health Organization.

Nilssen, O., & Cone, H. 1994. Screening patients for alcohol problems in primary health care settings. *Alcohol Health & Research World*, 18, 2: 136-139.

OPSS — Observatório Português dos Sistemas de Saúde. 2003. *SAÚDE: que rupturas?*. Lisboa: Escola Nacional de Saúde Pública.

Osuna Rodrigues, Jacinto. 1991. *Métodos de Muestreo.* Madrid: CIS, Centro de Investigaciones Sociológicas.

Osuna Rodrigues, Jacinto. 1993. *Métodos de Muestreo. Casos prácticos.* Madrid: CIS, Centro de Investigaciones Sociológicas.

Pinto, A. 2001. Álcool, entre o gosto e o desgosto, o drama português. *Cadernos de Bioética*, 25: 63-75.

Peretti-Watel, P., Beck, F., & Legleye, S. 2007. *Les Usages sociaux des drogues. Le lien social*. Paris: Presses Universitaires de France. http://catalogue.bnf.fr/ark:/12148/cb41001360j.

Petitat, André. 2014. *Secret et formes sociales*. Sociologie. Paris: P.U.F.

Petitat, André. n.d. *Secret et morphogenèse sociale*. Lausanne.

Petitat, André. 1996. Secret, représentation et normativité. In *Le Secret – Ethique, transparence et confidentialité*, Chaiers ER, 36. Lausanne: Université de Lausanne.

Piaser, Antonio, & Ladrière, Jean. 1976. *Pour une sociologie scientifique : épistémologie comparée de l'analyse conceptuelle préface de J. Ladrière. Interaction*. Paris La Haye: Mouton. http://catalogue.bnf.fr/ark:/12148/cb34694400w.

Poe, Edgar Alan. 2011. *A Carta Roubada*. São Paulo, Brasil: Panda Books.

Rehm, J., and Gadenne, V. 1990. *Intuitive Predictions and Professional Forecasts: Cognitive Processes and Social Consequences*. Oxford: Pergamon Press.

Rehm, J., Rehn, N., Room, R., Monteiro, M., Gmel, G., Jernigan, D. and Frick, U. 2003. The global distribution of average volume of alcohol consumption and patterns of drinking. *European Addiction Research* 9, 147-156.

Rehm, J., Klotsche, J. and Patra, J. 2007. Comparative quantification of alcohol exposure as risk factor for global burden of disease. International Journal of Methods in Psychiatric Research 16(2): 66–76.

Rehm, Jürgen e Emanuele Scafato. 2011. Indicators of alcohol consumption and attributable harm for monitoring and surveillance in European Union countries. *Addiction*, 106(1): 4-10.

Rehm, Jürgen, Kevin D. Shield, Maximilien X. Rehm, Gerrit Gmel, Ulrich Frick. 2012. *Alcohol consumption, alcohol dependence, and attributable burden of disease in Europe: Potential gains from effective interventions for alcohol dependence*. Toronto, Canada: Centre for Addiction and Mental Health.

Rehm, Jürgen, Shalini Kailasapillai, Elisabeth Larsen, Maximilien X. Rehm, Andriy V. Samokhvalov, Kevin D. Shield, Michael Roerecke, Dirk W. Lachenmeier. 2014. A systematic review of the epidemiology of unrecorded alcohol consumption and the chemical composition of unrecorded alcohol. *Addiction*, 109(6): 880-893.

Remy, Jean. 2005. Négociations et transaction sociale. *Négociations* 1,3: 81-95. https://doi.org/10.3917/neg.003.0081.

Remy, Jean. 2015. *L'Espace, un objet central de la sociologie*. Toulouse : Editions Érès.

Remy, J., Voyé, L., & Servais, E. 1978. *Produire ou reproduire?* Bruxelles: Vie ouvrière.

Robins, L.N., Wing, J., Wittchen, H.-U., Helzer, J.E., Babor, T.F., Burke, J., Farmer, A., Jablensky, A., Pickens, R., Regier, D.A., Sartorius, N., & Towle, L.H. 1989. The composite international diagnostic interview: An epidemiologic instrument suitable for use in conjunction with different diagnostic systems and in different cultures. *Archives of General Psychiatry*, 45, 1069-1077.

http://pubs.niaaa.nih.gov/publications/AssessingAlcohol/InstrumentPDFs/20_CIDI.pdf.

Saunders, J.B., Aasland, O.G., Babor, T.F., De La Fuente, J.R., & Grant, M. 1993. Development of the Alcohol Use Disorders Identification Test (AUDIT): WHO Collaborative Project on Early Detection of Persons with Harmful Alcohol Consumption-II. *Addiction* 88(6): 791-804.

Schröder, J. 2016. Face-to-face surveys. In *GESIS Survey Guidelines*, 7. Mannheim, Germany: GESIS – Leibniz Institute for the Social Sciences. https://doi.org/10.15465/gesis-sg_en_005.

Sierosławski, J., Foster, J., & Moskalewicz, J. 2013. Survey of European drinking surveys. Alcohol survey experiences of 22 European countries. *Drugs: Education, Prevention and Policy* 20,5, 383-398.

Sierosławski, J. 2011. Estimating annual alcohol consumption and analysis of drinking pattern. In J. Moskalewicz (ed.), *Pilot Drinking Survey Report*. Warsaw: Institute of Psychiatry and Neurology. http://www.alcsmart.ipin.edu.pl/files/smart_pilot_final_report. pdf, 16–34.

Simpura, Jussi e Thomas Karlsson. 2001. Trends in drinking patterns among adult population in 15 European countries, 1950 to 2000: a review. *Nordic Studies on Alcohol and Drugs*, 18(1): 31-53.

Smart *et al*. 1991. Use of the CAGE scale in a population survey of drinking. *Journal of Studies on Alcohol and Drugs*, Vol. 52, Issue 6.

Smith, Allan 'Ben', Madeleine King, Phyllis Butow e Ian Olver. 2013. A comparison of data quality and practicality of online versus postal questionnaires in a sample of testicular cancer survivors. *Psycho-Oncology*, 22(1): 233-237.

Sordo, L., Barrio, G., Bravo, M., Villalbí, J., Espelt, A., Neira, M., & Regidor, H. 2016. Estimating average alcohol consumption in the population using multiple sources: the case of Spain. *Population Health Metrics*. June 14: 21.

Steeh, C.G. 1981. Trends in nonresponse rates, 1952-1979. *Public Opinion Quarterly*, Vol. 45, 40-57. http://www.jstor.org/stable/2748317.

Thompson, M.E., Huang, Y.C., Boudreau, C., Fong, G., van den Putte, B., Nagelhout, G.E., & Willemsen, M.C. 2013. Accounting for the Effects of Data Collection Method Application to the International Tobacco Control Netherlands Survey. *Population*, 68(3).

Vannette, David L., & Krosnick, Jon A. 2013. *Answering Questions: A Comparison of Survey Satisficing and Mindlessness*. EUA: Stanford University.

Wallace, Paul. 2001. Patients with alcohol problems – Simple questioning is the key to effective identification and management. *The British Journal of General Practice*. Vol.51(464): 172-173.

Walsh, Brendan M., Grant, Marcus & World Health Organization. 1985. *Public health implications of alcohol production and trade*. Geneva: World Health Organization.
https://apps.who.int/iris/handle/10665/39696

Weisburd, D., & Britt, C. 2014. *Statistics in Criminal Justice*. New York: Springer.

Winter, Marielle de, Cohen, Peter, & Langemijer, Marieke. 1999. *Project to co-ordinate a methodological study to compare the prevalence of self-reported drug use in general population surveys*, OEDT project CT.97. EP.02. Lisbon: EMCDDA.

Wittchen, H.U., Robins, L.N., Cottler, L.B., Sartorius, N., Burke, J.D., & Regier, D. 1991. Clinical cross-cultural feasibility: reliability and sources of variance of the CIDI. *British Journal of Psychiatry*. 159: 645-53.

Wittchen, H.U. 1994. Reliability and validity studies of the WHO Composite International Diagnostic Interview (CIDI): A critical review. *Journal of Psychiatric Research*, 28, 57-84.

World Health Organization. 1992. *The ICD-10 Classification of Mental and Behavioural Disorders: Clinical descriptions and diagnostic guidelines*. Geneve: WHO.

World Health Organization. Programme on Substance Abuse. 1994. *International profile: alcohol and other drugs 1994* / compiled by Bob Williams et al. Alcoholism and Drug Addiction Research Foundation.

World Health Organization. 2000. *International guide for monitoring alcohol consumption and related harm*. Geneva: Department of Mental Health and Substance Dependence, Noncommunicable Diseases and Health. WHO Publication Number WHO/MSD/MSB/00.4.

World Health Organization. 2004. *Global Status Report on Alcohol*. Geneve: World Health Organization.

World Health Organization. 2010. *Global strategy to reduce the harmful use of alcohol*. Geneve: World Health Organization.
World Health Organization. 2014. *Global Status Report on Alcohol and Health 2014*. Geneve: World Health Organization.
World Health Organization. 2018. *Global Status Report on Alcohol and Health 2018*. Geneve: World Health Organization.